MW01267983

Hearing instrument technology
A. Vonlanthen

ISBN-Nr.: 3-274-00089-2

Hearing instrument technology

for the hearing healthcare professional

A. Vonlanthen

Foreword

This book began to take shape while I was teaching trainee hearing instrument acousticians. A special feature of the program I was involved in is that it is a part-time, designed for working adults. Their technical knowledge varies considerably and depends largely on their previous training. From a teaching point of view, the main challenge was to give students the necessary basic know-how during the first part of the course. We would then build on this during the second phase and provide them with all the knowledge they would need subsequently, in their chosen profession.

This essentially "back-to-basics" approach may well be advantageous for acousticians in other countries with different training systems.

This was one of the reasons why Phonak supported this project from the very beginning. Needless to say, the course itself is neutral in content and can be used in any situation.

The author would particularly like to thank Sonja Krienbühl whose commitment and precision were invaluable in preparing the charts for publication. The layout, make-up and editing were in the capable hands of Andrea Gnädinger. A special word of thanks also goes to the translator of the English version, who has made the book available to a much wider audience.

A. Vonlanthen, December 1995

Table of Contents

1 Introduction

Hearing instruments are sound amplifiers. Their function is to amplify sound to a level such that a hearing-impaired person can both detect and, most importantly, make effective use of the acoustic signal (Acoustical technology; 1. Veit [14]).

Although this is certainly the primary function of a hearing instrument, the different degrees and etiologies of hearing impairment and associated problems place varying demands on them. A complete description of hearing loss which takes into account not only the audiogram configuration, but also the nature and degree of the associated problems, has not previously been possible. Despite the last few years' enormous progress in hearing instrument technology, it is still only possible to provide some help in the case of hearing loss, but not to correct for it. In this book, hearing instrument technology will be comprehensively reviewed, ending with a brief discussion of the direction it will take in the future.

1.1 Historical overview

The development of hearing instrument technology can be divided into 5 phases. There is some overlap between these phases. The intervals shown in Figure 1.1 are intended to give a general impression of the time period for each phase.

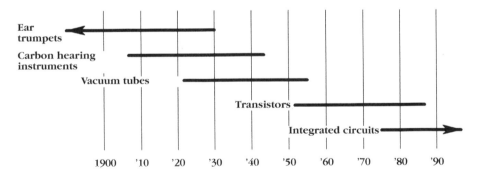

Figure 1.1: The 5 phases of development of hearing instrument technology

The first phase was an (mechanical) acoustic phase in which acoustic amplification was achieved by means of different types of ear trumpets. The first of man's hearing instruments was a hand cupped behind the ear. (Unfortunately, this is still the most common means of assisting hearing). Figure 1.2 illustrates how a hand cupped behind the ear changes the acoustics of the signal. There is a resonance with an amplitude of approximately 10 dB between 1 and 2 kHz. At higher frequencies, there is actually an attenuation of the signal. (Note: the diagram represents an insertion gain measurement. The reader is referred to Chapter 3.3.2 for a discussion of insertion gain.)

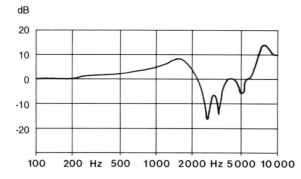

Figure 1.2: The insertion gain from a hand held behind the ear

At the beginning of the 19th century, various kinds and shapes of ear trumpets were produced. A significant amount of amplification could be achieved using an ear trumpet. (see Fig.1.4).

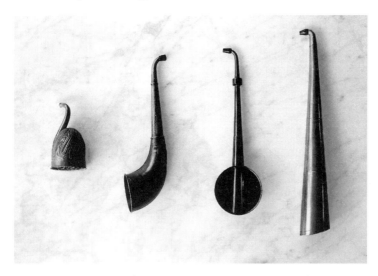

Figure 1.3: Various types of ear trumpets

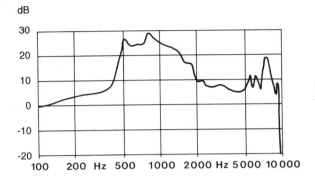

Figure 1.4: The insertion gain of an ear trumpet

It was clear that a stereophonic arrangement would be optimal!

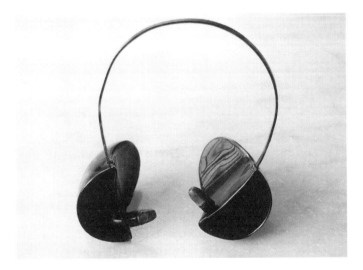

Figure 1.5: Ear trumpets for a stereophonic fitting (1930)

The second phase in the development of hearing instrument technology took place in the early part of the twentieth century. In this phase, telephone technology was used in developing hearing instruments. The problems with carbon hearing instruments were twofold: first, the large distortion produced through the resonances of the microphone and the receiver and, second, excessive noise from the microphone.

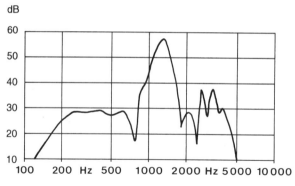

Figure 1.6: The frequency response of a carbon hearing instrument

Figure 1.7 shows a carbon hearing instrument from 1922 with a microphone (large capsule) and ear receiver. The batteries required are not shown.

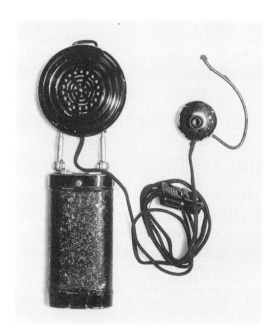

Figure 1.7: Carbon hearing instrument

In the third phase, vacuum tubes were utilized in the construction of hearing instruments. This made a much greater acoustic amplification possible than with the carbon hearing instruments.

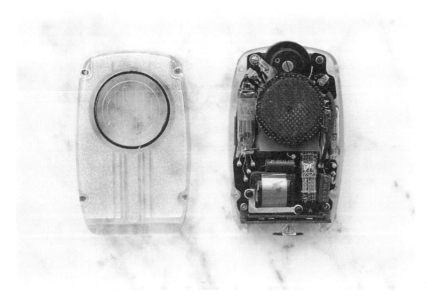

Figure 1.8: A body hearing instrument with three vacuum tubes (1939)

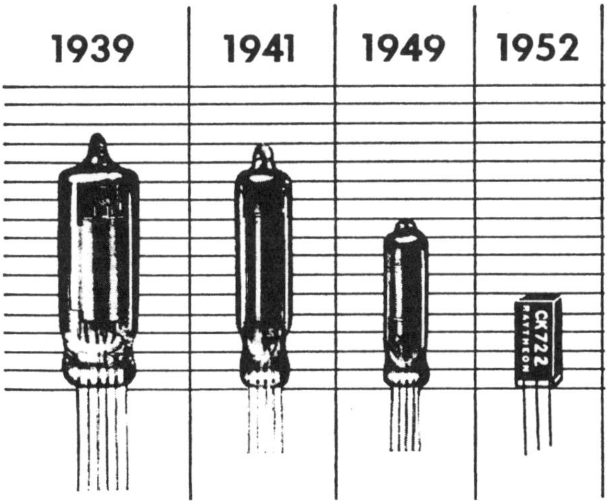

Figure 1.9: Development from vacuum tubes to the transistor
(Berger [2])

The development of the transistor led hearing instrument technology into the fourth phase. Vacuum tubes were replaced by much smaller transistors, making it possible to produce hearing instruments that could be worn on the head.

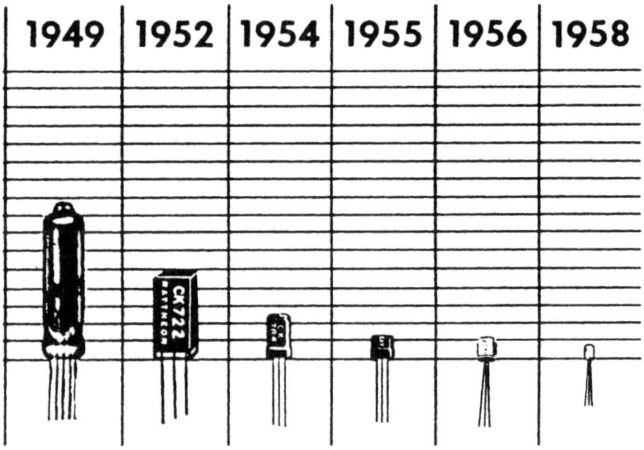

1949	1952	1954	1955	1956	1958

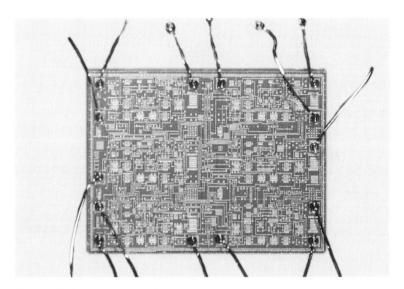

Figure 1.10: Further development of transistors (Berger [2])

Today, we are in the fifth phase in which transistors have been integrated, enabling the production of hearing instruments with over 1000 transistors.

Figure 1.11: An integrated circuit

1.2 Basic components of a hearing instrument

The assembly of a hearing instrument is fundamentally the same whether it is a behind-the-ear, in-the-ear, eyeglass or body hearing instrument.

A hearing instrument consists of:

microphone:	transduces acoustic signals into electrical signals.
amplifier:	amplifies the electrical signal.
battery:	supplies power to the hearing instrument.
user controls:	influence the operation of the hearing instrument. Can be changed by the user of the hearing instrument and/or the hearing healthcare professional.
receiver:	converts the electrical signal back into an acoustic signal.

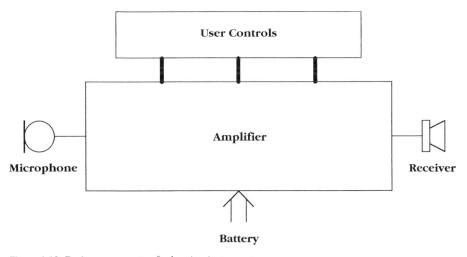

Figure 1.12: Basic components of a hearing instrument

1.3 Basic components of a behind-the-ear hearing instrument

In order to facilitate a better understanding of a hearing instrument, the construction of a behind-the-ear unit is examined in detail here. The illustration in Figure 1.13 will be employed to bring out certain concepts of hearing instrument technology.

Transducers
The acoustic heart of a hearing instrument. Because of the space available in a behind-the-ear unit, particularly good results can be achieved with a careful choice of transducers.

Control elements
The volume control and M/T switch are control elements which are manipulated by the user. Trimmers are the control elements which the hearing healthcare professional sets appropriately for the individual hearing loss during fitting. The modern programmable hearing instruments are set by means of a computer instead of trimmers. The trimmers on the instrument are replaced by a small programming socket by which the instrument is connected to the computer via a cable.

Amplifier
The amplifier constitutes the electronics of the hearing instrument and consists of various circuit elements. The amplifier is fed the signal from the microphone, amplifies it according to the settings, and sends the appropriately amplified signal on to the receiver.

Acoustic modifications
It is often quite simple to alter the output signal by means of acoustic modifications. In this way, the hearing healthcare professional can make significant improvements in the fitting of a hearing instrument.

Accessories
Accessories are all items which can be used along with the hearing instrument.

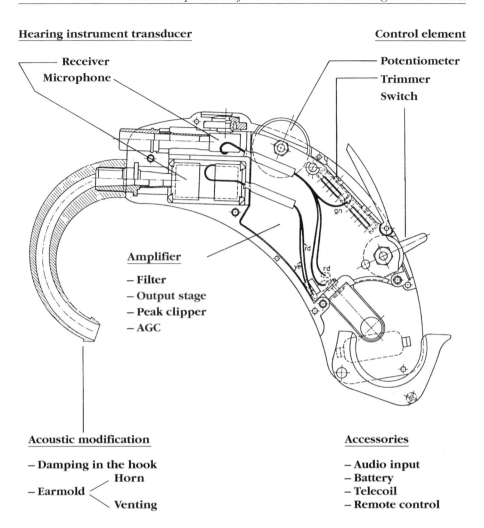

Hearing instrument transducer

Receiver
Microphone

Control element

Potentiometer
Trimmer
Switch

Amplifier

– Filter
– Output stage
– Peak clipper
– AGC

Acoustic modification

– Damping in the hook
Horn
– Earmold
Venting

Accessories

– Audio input
– Battery
– Telecoil
– Remote control

Figure 1.13: Basic components of a BTE hearing instrument

2 Hearing instrument types

2.1 Body hearing instrument

The body hearing instrument is the oldest form of construction for an electronic hearing instrument. The microphone and the amplifier circuit, together with all the user and fitter controls are in a housing which is normally carried on the body or in a pocket. The receiver (earphone) is inserted in the ear and connected to the main unit by a cord.

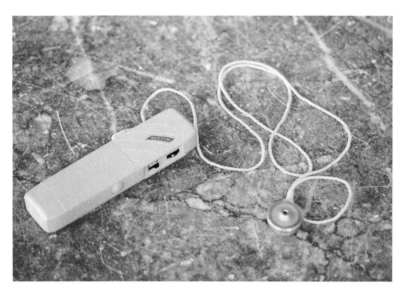

Figure 2.1: Body hearing instrument

Although the market share of the body unit is steadily becoming smaller, it is, in certain cases, advantageous compared to other types of hearing instruments.

Advantages and disadvantages of body units

+ A body hearing instrument offers the greatest possible acoustic amplification due to the maximal distance between the receiver and the microphone.
+ Body hearing instruments have large user controls which make them easy to operate for those with poor manual dexterity.
+ Body hearing instruments offer the greatest maximum output sound pressure level due to the earphone.
+ Body hearing instruments are cost-effective as they use large batteries.
+ In the case of bone conduction receivers, the body hearing instrument offers the advantage of there being no mechanical feedback.

In addition to being cosmetically unappealing, the body hearing instrument has the following significant disadvantages:

– Its cumbersome size, as well as the one or two cords connecting the instrument to the receiver, make it awkward to wear.
– The microphone is not on the head, precluding directional and stereophonic hearing.
– Clothing rubbing against the microphone results in amplified noise.

dB Gain

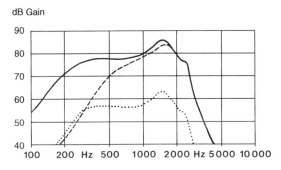

dB SPL Output

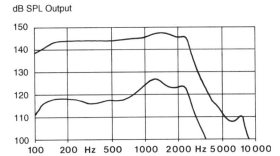

Figure 2.2: The gain and output frequency responses of a body hearing instrument (Ear simulator measurements)

2.2 Eyeglass hearing instrument

The first eyeglass hearing instruments were produced in the early fifties.
In the eyeglass hearing instrument, all of the components are built into the bows of the eyeglass frame.
The inlet for the microphone is located either at the hinge or behind the ear. The further forward the microphone inlet is located, the less is the danger of feedback. However, the directional hearing of the wearer suffers with a forward placement of the microphone.
The receivers are at the nonhinged ends of the bows and are joined to the earmold by plastic tubing.

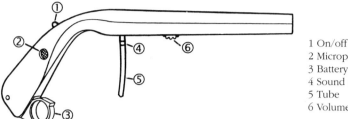

1 On/off switch
2 Microphone inlet
3 Battery compartment
4 Sound outlet
5 Tube
6 Volume control

Figure 2.3: The eyeglass hearing instrument

Advantages of eyeglass hearing instruments

+ They are ideal when using bone conduction receivers.
+ Eyeglass hearing instruments are preferred for CROS applications since the wires can be mounted in the bows of the frame.
+ In the case of an open ear fitting, it is possible to mount the microphone right at the front (near the hinge) so as to have as large a distance as possible between the microphone and the receiver, resulting in less feedback.

Disadvantages

– Creating an interdependency between hearing and seeing is undesirable. With eyeglass hearing instruments the person cannot hear when they remove their eyeglasses. Likewise, the wearer must do without his eyeglasses if the hearing instrument needs repair. In the case of loss, the person loses both hearing instrument and optical correction.
– Conventional eyeglass hearing instruments are very heavy and seldom considered cosmetically acceptable.

Today, hearing instruments built into eyeglass frame bows are rarely fitted. Instead a behind-the-ear instrument can be mounted on the bow of the glasses by means of an adaptor. This is often an attractive solution, especially in the case of an open ear fitting.

The result is both elegant and inconspicuous since there is only a small length of tubing from the bow of the glasses to the ear canal and no earmold. Statistics show that a BTE instrument is preferred for open ear fittings. Figure 2.4 shows the ideal in elegance and discretion for a hearing instrument with a spectacles adaptor.

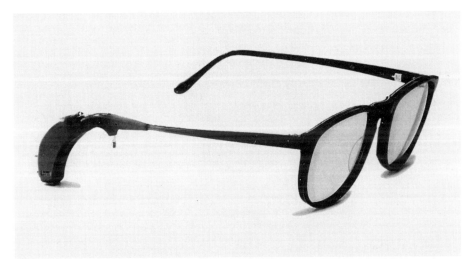

Figure 2.4: A combination hearing instrument and spectacles

2.3 Behind-the-ear hearing instrument

Today the behind-the-ear hearing instrument is the most frequently used hearing instrument in Europe. The receiver, microphone and amplifier are built into a housing which is worn behind the ear. Sound is carried via soft plastic tubing to the ear canal.

Over the last 30 years, several different types of behind-the-ear hearing instruments have been developed. In the first generation of behind-the-ear hearing instruments, great care was taken to place the microphone and receiver as far from each other as possible. The reason for this was mechanical and acoustic feedback. Behind-the-ear hearing instruments were also constructed with external receivers (these were built into the earmold to obtain a better acoustic transmission), but the electrical connection between the receiver and amplifier failed to meet the mechanical demands. Figure 2.5 shows how the components typically have been arranged in a behind-the-ear hearing instrument up to now.

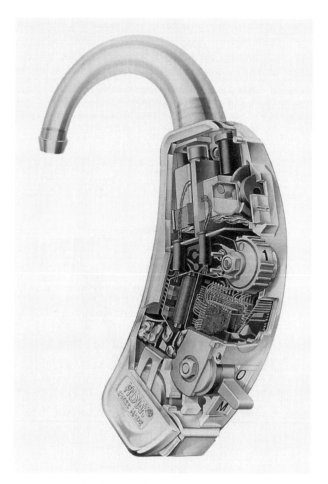

Figure 2.5: A behind-the-ear hearing instrument

Advantages of a BTE hearing instrument

+ Open ear fittings are possible.
+ Directional microphones can be utilized.
+ A BTE represents a good compromise between the more powerful but large and unwieldy body hearing unit and the smaller but less powerful in-the-ear unit.
+ BTE instruments are inconspicuous.
+ The BTE hearing instrument has a housing which is roomy enough to accomodate new technological developments.
+ Possibility of including the best acoustic transducers.

Disadvantages of the behind-the-ear hearing instrument

– Resonance of the soft plastic tubing negatively affects natural sound quality.
– The microphone is not in the ear.
– It is not viable to use bone conduction receivers.

dB Gain

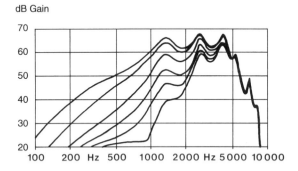

dB SPL Output

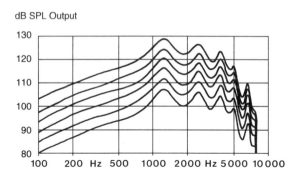

Figure 2.6: The gain and output frequency responses of a behind-the-ear hearing instrument (measured in a 2 cc coupler)

2.4 In-the-ear hearing instrument

In the case of in-the-ear hearing instruments, the components are all built into a housing which fits into the concha or ear canal.
Today, there are two types of ITE units which differ in their construction

a) The custom ITE hearing instrument

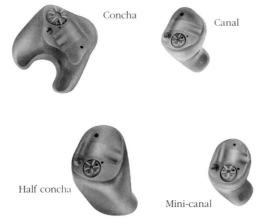

Concha

Canal

Half concha

Mini-canal

Figure 2.7: Custom ITE hearing instruments

b) The (Semi-) modular instrument

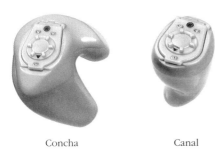

Figure 2.8: Modular hearing instruments

Concha   Canal

a) In the case of the custom ITE, a shell is first produced from an impression of the user's ear and the components built into the shell. The receiver is placed as deep in the ear canal as possible, while the microphone is positioned in the concha. The amplifier, battery and potentiometer are then installed in the shell wherever there is enough space.

b) Modular ITE instruments are built into a standard housing which is then attached to a custom earmold. In a semi-modular unit, the receiver is installed in the custom earmold.

A custom ITE is advantageous in that it makes optimal use of the entire space occupied by the shell. A custom ITE is the smallest form of hearing instrument. The advantage of a modular unit is that it is manufactured to more exact specifications, resulting in better quality control (fewer rejects).

Advantages and disadvantages of in-the-ear hearing instruments (custom-built or modular)

+ Acoustically, ITE instruments are superior to other types. The microphone is situated within the ear, thereby taking advantage of the pinna's function. The receiver is located as near the tympanic membrane as possible, resulting in enhancement of high frequency information due to the small cavity enclosed by the instrument.
+ ITE instruments are inconspicuous.
+ ITE instruments are generally comfortable to wear.
− Acoustic feedback is more likely to be a problem, especially with the high levels of amplification required in the case of more severe hearing losses.
− The small size of ITE instruments often necessitates compromises in construction at the cost of sound quality. There is simply not space enough for good electronics.
− ITE instruments are less durable than other types.
− ITE hearing instruments are frequently defective because of the intrusion of debris.
− The small batteries necessitate frequent battery changes.
− ITE instruments are frequently tight-fitting due to space limitations. This results in reduced wearer comfort due to occlusion.

dB Gain

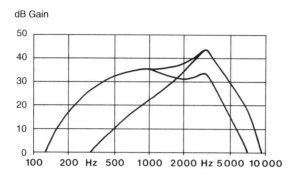

dB SPL Output

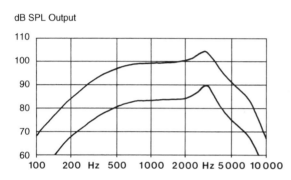

Figure 2.9: The gain and output frequency responses of an in-the-ear unit (2 cc coupler measurement)

2.5 Statistics on the types of hearing instruments

It is interesting to study the distribution of the types of hearing instruments used today.

The trend is towards increasingly smaller units, that is, to in-the-ear units.
In 1977, Werner Güttner (Hörgerätetechnik [6]) wrote:
With the arrival of the in-the-ear hearing instrument in 1965, the market share of this group of hearing instruments was 2%. Thereafter, it fell steadily until it reached 0.3% in 1972. Today, in 1977, hardly anyone orders this kind of hearing instrument in Germany.
One reason for this was that size constraints made it necessary to use small acoustic transducers which were poor in quality. Another reason was the limited amplification due to acoustic feedback problems.

There are two main reasons for the subsequent success of the in-the-ear units:
a) The rapid development of electronic and acoustic transducers over the last 15 years has made it possible to produce higher fidelity ITE instruments than ever before.

b) An inconspicuous hearing instrument is often more appealing to the wearer.

In contrast to the USA, behind-the-ear hearing instruments are still preferred in Europe. It is, however, only a matter of time before ITE units conquer the market as has been the case in the USA.

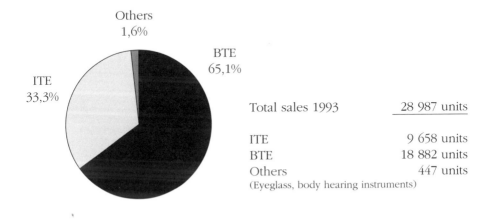

Total sales 1993   <u>28 987 units</u>

ITE   9 658 units
BTE   18 882 units
Others   447 units
(Eyeglass, body hearing instruments)

Figure 2.10: The market share of different hearing instrument types in Switzerland (1993)

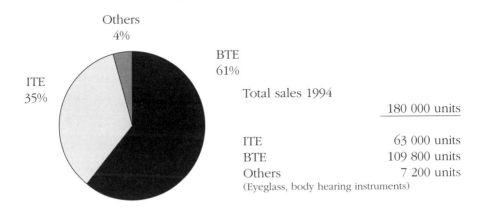

Total sales 1994

<u>180 000 units</u>

ITE   63 000 units
BTE   109 800 units
Others   7 200 units
(Eyeglass, body hearing instruments)

Figure 2.11: The market share of different hearing instrument types in France (1994)

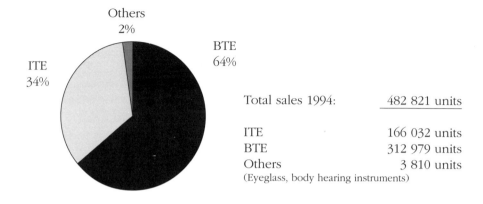

Figure 2.12: The market share of different hearing instrument types in Germany (1994)

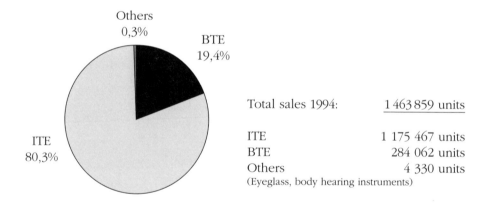

Figure 2.13: The market share of different hearing instrument types in the USA (1994)

3 Hearing instrument measurements and standards

The first means of assessing hearing instruments was the human ear. The hearing instrument was designed, tested and modified dependent on either the developer's or the user's judgments. A trained ear is, in fact, quite fast and accurate in assessing the quality of a hearing instrument. However, in order to describe and evaluate the transmission characteristics of hearing instruments and enable comparison with one another, it was necessary to develop objective measuring methods. It was agreed that only a few easily measured physical parameters would constitute standard testing of hearing instruments. The data obtained by such testing differs from measurements made at the user's tympanic membrane, but have the advantage of being easily controlled and reproducible. In order to measure a hearing instrument, certain requirements must be satisfied.

1) Free field measurement

The data obtained measuring a hearing instrument in a normal room will be confounded by the reflection of sound from the walls. Furthermore, such reverberation would make comparisons with data obtained elsewhere impossible.
→ Hearing instruments must be measured in free field!
Ideally, an anechoic chamber would be used, but such rooms are large and expensive. Small sound-treated boxes have been developed which are sufficiently free of reflection in the hearing instrument frequency range (100 Hz to 10 kHz) to make them appropriate for measurement of hearing instruments. Figure 3.1 shows a sound box, unique in design, but rather expensive.

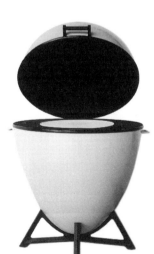

Figure 3.1: Brüel & Kjær (B&K) sound box

2) Linear loudspeaker frequency response

Any nonlinearity in the loudspeaker frequency response in the sound box causes errors in the measurement of the hearing instrument frequency response.
Therefore, the frequency response of the loudspeaker must be flat (± 1 dB) between 100 Hz and 10 kHz. As no loudspeaker (in the normal price range) can
offer such an accurate frequency response, the nonlinearity in the loudspeaker's
frequency response is compensated for electronically.
This is accomplished as follows:

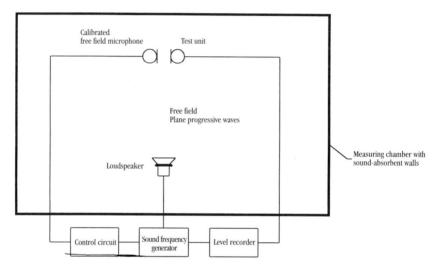

Figure 3.2: Basic structure of a controlled sound box

A control microphone (a second microphone) is installed in the sound box symmetrically opposite the test point. The control microphone measures the sound
pressure.
Whenever the sound pressure diverges from the reference value, then electrical
input to the loudspeaker amplifier is rapidly adjusted so that the sound pressure at the control microphone again matches the reference value.

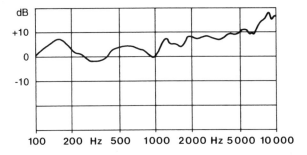

Figure 3.3: Frequency response of a loudspeaker in the sound box (not controlled)

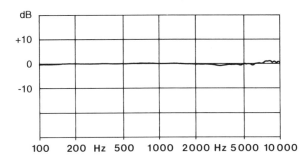

Figure 3.4: Controlled frequency response of the loudspeaker in the sound box

There is a second method of achieving a linear frequency response in the sound box. The substitution method.

This method is particulary favored for clinical use by hearing healthcare professionals. Only one microphone is required for the substitution method. It differs from the comparison method in that the electrical input to the loudspeaker amplifier needed to achieve the desired sound pressure is determined in advance of measuring the hearing instrument.

Prior to measuring any hearing instruments, the loudspeaker frequency response is determined with the measuring microphone at the test point. This curve is stored and the microphone is removed.

During subsequent measurments of hearing instruments, the electrical input to the loudspeaker amplifier is manipulated so as to "flatten out" the stored curve. Thus, if the stored curve has a 5 dB notch at 10 kHz, then the electrical input to the loudspeaker amplifier is increased so as to give a 5 dB more intense signal at this frequency. Likewise, a 7 dB spike at 6 kHz would be compensated for by a corresponding decrease in the input to the loudspeaker amplifer, resulting in a 7 dB less intense signal at this frequency. In this way, a linear frequency response is achieved.

3.1 Hearing instrument coupler and ear simulator

Ideally, a hearing instrument would be measured in the ear to assess its actual performance. However, this would be costly and, due to the nonstandard nature of human ears, would make impossible any meaningful comparison of results. Thus, analyses of hearing instruments are made using standardized "artificial ears," which have been designed to approximate the acoustic characteristics of an average ear.

A coupler is a device connecting a receiver and a measuring microphone. It contains an air-filled chamber with a given shape. This serves to load the receiver. *Couplers* do not imitate the equivalent volume of the human ear. The acoustic impedance of a coupler is different from that of the natural ear.

The sound from the receiver is measured in the coupler with a microphone.

In 1959, a coupler for hearing instruments was specified as having a chamber with an effective volume of 2 ccm (old IEC standard).

Ear simulators take into account the equivalent volumes or loading of the receiver of the hearing instrument with the same average frequency-dependent impedance of the human ear in the hearing frequency range. This ensures that the sound pressure which the measuring microphone picks up agrees with the average value present at the eardrum.

3.1.1 The 2 cc coupler

An electroacoustic coupler with a cavity of 2 ccm is used in place of the human ear for the measurements described above. At one end of the cavity is a capacitor microphone which transforms sounds into electrical signals that are supplied to the measuring instruments.

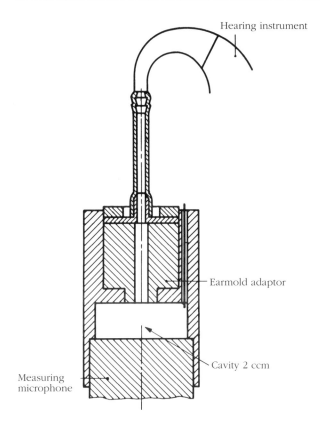

Figure 3.5: 2 cc coupler for behind-the-ear hearing instrument measurements

The means for mounting the hearing instrument on the coupler is modified according to the type of hearing instrument (e.g. behind-the-ear or in-the-ear).
In Figure 3.5, one can see how the connection between the coupler and the behind-the-ear unit is effected via a length of tubing. This tubing should have a length of 25 mm and an inner diameter of 2 mm.
For an in-the-ear unit, where the receiver is in the ear canal, the arrangement should be as shown in Figure 3.6.

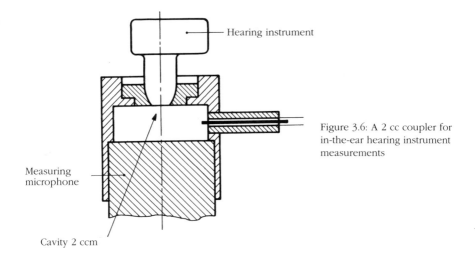

— Hearing instrument

Figure 3.6: A 2 cc coupler for
in-the-ear hearing instrument
measurements

Measuring
microphone

Cavity 2 ccm

Typical hearing instrument curves as measured with the 2 cc coupler are shown
in Figures 3.7, 3.8, 3.9 and 3.10.

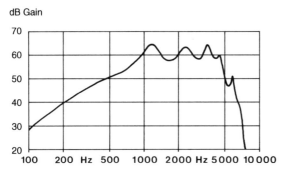

dB Gain

Figure 3.7: The gain response of a
behind-the-ear unit measured with
the 2 cc coupler

dB SPL Output

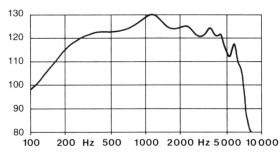

Figure 3.8: The maximum power output response of a behind-the-ear unit measured with the 2 cc coupler

dB Gain

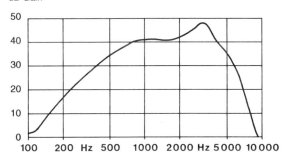

Figure 3.9: The gain response of an in-the-ear unit measured with the 2 cc coupler

dB SPL Output

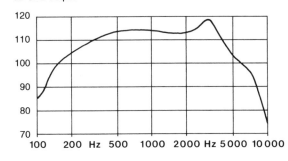

Figure 3.10: The maximum power output response of an in-the-ear unit measured with the 2 cc coupler

The average human ear has a volume considerably smaller than 2 ccm. As a consequence, measurements made in the 2 cc coupler differ markedly from those made in the ear, particulary at frequencies higher than 1 kHz.
In this case, the SPL measured in the 2 cc coupler will be too low compared to real ear measurements. This was the impetus behind the 1981 issuance of a new IEC standard for a better coupler.
Since the acoustical properties of this new coupler more closely approximated those of the human ear, it was called an EAR SIMULATOR. It is manufactured by Brüel and Kjær (B&K) in Denmark.
Although the ear simulator has been on the market for a long time, there are some countries (e.g. the USA) which still use the 2 cc coupler as a standard (ANSI Standard).
The reasons for the continued worldwide use of the 2 cc coupler (among hearing healthcare professionals) include the reproducibility of results, ease of use and relative economy.

3.1.2 The ear simulator from B&K (B&K ear simulator)

In 1971, the members of the working group 'Artificial Ear for Insert Earphones' in the IEC (International Electrotechnical Commission) ratified the following required properties for an ear simulator:

– The materials used should be mechanically stable and easy to manufacture.
– The simulator should have a geometrical similarity to the ear canal.
– The smallest frequency range measurable should be 80–6000 Hz, extensible, if possible, to 10 kHz.
– The acoustic impedance should be the same as the corresponding mean value of the human ear.
– The transmission constant of the different kinds of hearing instruments should correspond to the mean value measured at the real eardrum.

In the late seventies, the company Brüel and Kjær (B&K) developed an ear simulator which was selected by the IEC as the standard for hearing instrument measurements. In 1981, this was encompassed in the new IEC Standard.

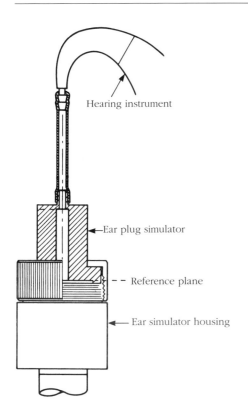

Hearing instrument

Ear plug simulator

Reference plane

Ear simulator housing

Figure 3.11: B&K ear simulator for behind-the-ear hearing instruments [3]

The B&K ear simulator is primarily intended for the measurement of hearing instruments which are coupled to the ear via tubing, earmolds, etc. It has therefore been designed to fulfill the requirements of the proposed IEC and ANSI standards for an ear simulator for measuring hearing instruments.

The ear simulator closely reproduces the physical parameters of the human ear, presenting the hearing instrument under test with an impedance approximating that of the real human ear.

The ear simulator consists of a main housing into which are assembled a number of rings forming annular volumes of air connected to the main cavity of the housing by air passages. The main canal volume is similar in shape and volume to that of the human ear and provides a similar acoustic impedance to the hearing instrument being tested. The pressure microphone is screwed directly into the housing of the ear simulator.

The ear simulator, like the 2 cc coupler, can also be modified to suit different hearing instruments. The various adaptors supplied with the ear simulator allow simple mounting of all types of hearing instruments.

The hearing instrument should always be placed flush with the reference plane of the ear simulator in order to obtain the best reproducibility of the measurements.

The earmold adaptor for external receivers and the ear adaptor for behind-the-ear units can automatically be aligned correctly reference plane. Figures 3.11/3.12/3.13 show the methods for mounting the various types of hearing instruments to the ear simulator with the adaptors provided.

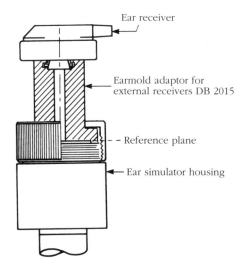

Ear receiver

Earmold adaptor for external receivers DB 2015

- - Reference plane

Ear simulator housing

Figure 3.12: Mounting of a button type receiver on the ear simulator [3]

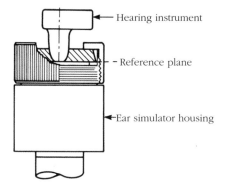

Hearing instrument

- Reference plane

Ear simulator housing

Figure 3.13: Mounting of an in-the-ear instrument with a shaped earmold on the ear simulator [3]

Calibration

Accuracy in hearing instrument measurments require occasional calibration of the ear simulator (or 2 cc coupler). This can be done most easily using the B&K pistonphone. The pistonphone is connected directly to the ear simulator and provides a stable 250 Hz signal of 124 dB SPL. The measuring instrument (audiometer) must be adjusted to this 124 dB SPL signal. Figure 3.14 shows an ear simulator with the pistonphone connected.

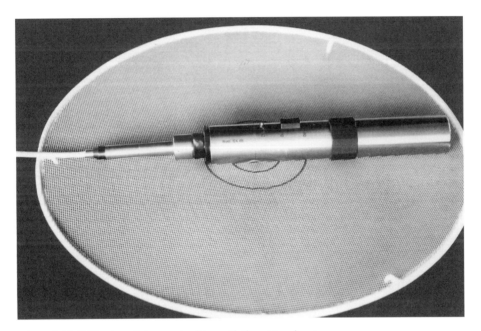

Figure 3.14: Calibration of the ear simulator with the pistonphone

Summary

The ear simulator was developed to resemble the complex auditory canal more closely than the 2 cc coupler. Ear simulator measurements correspond better on average with real ear measurements than those made in the 2 cc coupler. It must be stressed, however, that the ear simulator is an instrument, and that the measurements obtained with it can only be approximately related to an individual ear. The ear simulator is particularly suitable for comparing one hearing instrument with another, although this is also possible with the 2 cc coupler.

For the hearing healthcare professional, it is often confusing that some hearing instruments are measured with the ear simulator and others with the 2 cc coupler.

a) Comparative measurements of a behind-the-ear unit with an ear simulator and with a 2 cc coupler.

dB Gain

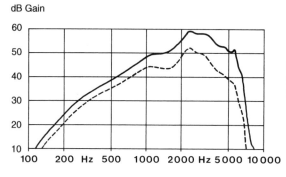

Figure 3.15: Gain response of a BTE measured with ear simulator (——) and 2 cc coupler (- - -)

dB SPL Output

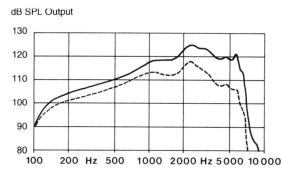

Figure 3.16: SSPL 90 response of a BTE measured with ear simulator (——) and 2 cc coupler (- - -)

b) Comparative measurements of an in-the-ear unit with an ear simulator and with a 2 cc coupler.

dB Gain

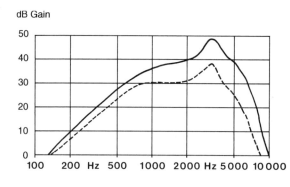

Figure 3.17: Gain response of an ITE measured with ear simulator (——) and 2 cc coupler (- - -)

dB SPL Output

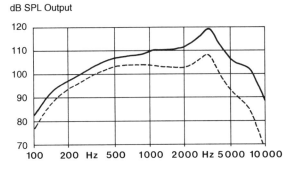

Figure 3.18: SSPL 90 response of a ITE measured with ear simulator (——) and 2 cc coupler (- - -)

It is clear from the comparative measurements that the sound pressure level in the ear simulator is up to 10 dB higher than in the 2 cc coupler.

The frequency response of a hearing instrument measured in an ear simulator will show more gain in the high frequency range than when a 2 cc coupler is used for the measurement.

One of the main advantages of the ear simulator is that the results obtained for high frequencies are more similar to real ear measurments than are those obtained with a 2 cc coupler. There are also differences in measurements made with an ear structural nature of the hearing instrument (behind-the-ear or in-the-ear).

3.2 Hearing instrument measurement in the sound box (in accordance with IEC 1983 [7])

Maximum acoustic gain, reference test gain, maximum output sound pressure level, etc., are all specific data for a hearing instrument which can be measured in a sound box.

This chapter describes the procedures and necessary instrumentation for performing such measurements.

The basis for these measurements is the new IEC standard 1983 (with B&K Ear-Simulator). Obtaining measurements in accordance with other standards and with other couplers (2 cc) will be covered in section [3.4].

The requirements for the measuring of the acoustic properties of a hearing instrument are summarized in Figure 3.19.

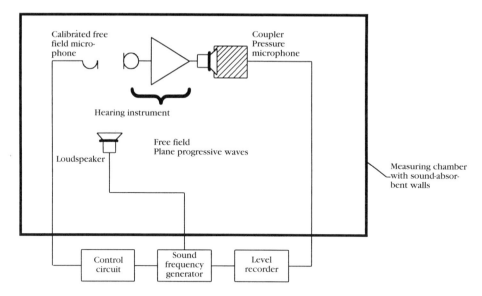

Figure 3.19: Basic test arrangement for hearing instruments

The sound box has sound-absorbent walls in order to maintain free field conditions.

An audio frequency generator drives a loudspeaker, which is also located in the sound box.

With this set-up, it is possible to use either the substitution or the comparison method as described at the beginning of this chapter. The comparison method will be utilized in the example.

The hearing instrument microphone and the control microphone (balanced in the free field) are near to one another and are symmetrically arranged with respect to the axis of the sound source.

The automatic control circuit which is regulated by the control microphone maintains the desired sound pressure level at the measuring point at the desired height while the frequency is altered.

The hearing instrument is connected to the ear simulator (or the coupler). The pressure microphone in the ear simulator is not subjected to the output sound level and passes the measured value to the level recorder. The paper drive of the level recorder and the frequency changes of the generator run synchronously.

Explanation of terms

In order to measure the hearing instrument accurately in the sound box and to enable comparison with other measurements (e.g. a data sheet), it is necessary to be familiar with certain terms.

Acoustic gain
The difference between the output sound pressure level developed in the ear simulator by the hearing instrument and the input sound pressure level measured at the test point.

Full on acoustic gain
The acoustic gain under essentially linear input/output conditions obtainable from the hearing instrument measured with the gain control at maximum (full-on) and at stated settings of the other hearing instrument controls.

Maximum saturation sound pressure level
The maximum value of a saturation sound pressure level frequency response curve produced in the ear simulator.

Output sound pressure level for an input sound pressure level of 90 dB SPL (OSPL 90 or SSPL 90)
The sound pressure level produced in the ear simulator with an input sound pressure level of 90 dB SPL, the gain control being in the full-on position and the other controls set for maximum gain. The abbreviation for this term is OSPL 90 (or OSPL 90 or SSPL 90 frequency response curve).

Reference test frequency
The frequency at which the setting of the gain control is made in relation to OSPL 90 to obtain a reference test position of the gain control. The reference test frequency is normally 1600 Hz. For certain hearing instruments, a higher reference test frequency is more appropriate (so called high-tone hearing instruments). In this case, 2500 Hz is used as the reference test frequency, and this should be clearly stated in the report.

Reference test gain control position
The setting of the hearing instrument gain control which provides an output sound pressure level in the ear simulator of 15±1 dB less than OSPL 90 for an input sound pressure level of 60 dB SPL at the reference test frequency. If the gain available will not permit this, full-on gain control position of the hearing instrument should be used.

Reference test gain
The acoustic gain of the hearing instrument at the reference test frequency with the setting of the gain control set to the reference test gain control position.

Basic frequency response curve
The frequency response curve obtained at the reference test gain setting with an input sound pressure level of 60 dB SPL.

We turn our attention now to the procedures involved in carrying out the measurements defined above.

3.2.1 Output sound pressure level frequency response for an input of 90 dB SPL.

The purpose of this test is to determine the sound pressure level obtained in the ear simulator when using an input of 90 dB SPL and the gain control in the full-on position as a function of frequency.

Test procedure:

a) Turn the gain control full on and set other controls to the required positions.

b) Adjust the input sound pressure level to 90 dB SPL at a suitable frequency.

c) Vary the frequency of the sound source over the recommended frequency range from 200 Hz to 8000 Hz keeping the input sound pressure level constant at 90 dB SPL. Record the sound pressure level in the ear simulator.

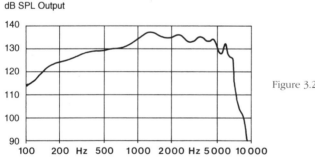

Figure 3.20: OSPL 90 curve

3.2.2 Full-on acoustic gain frequency response

The purpose of this test is to determine the full-on acoustic gain obtainable with the hearing instrument. The output sound pressure level in the ear simulator is measured at full-on gain control setting with an input below the hearing instrument's saturation sound pressure level.

Test procedure:

a) Turn the gain control full on and set other controls to the required positions.

b) At a suitable frequency, set the input sound pressure level so that it is below the hearing instrument's saturation sound pressure level, where the relationship between the level of the input and output is essentially linear. Such conditions are considered to exist if at all frequencies within the range of 200 Hz to 8000 Hz, a change of the input sound pressure level of 10 dB causes a change of recorded output level of 10±1 dB. The input sound pressure level must be reported.

c) The frequency response with full-on gain is measured by varying the frequency of the sound source over the recommended frequency range of 200 Hz to 8000 Hz, keeping the input sound pressure level constant.

d) The full-on acoustic gain is plotted as a function of frequency and may be reported for a specific frequency.

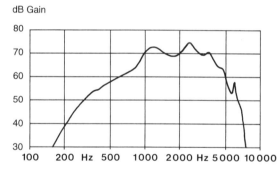

Figure 3.21: Full-on acoustic gain frequency response

3.2.3 Basic frequency response

The purpose of this test is to measure the frequency response of a hearing instrument without acoustic (feedback) or mechanical (vibration) problems.

Note: If one compares the shape of the full-on acoustic gain frequency response with the basic frequency response, then acoustic or mechanical problems can be identified. → The more similar the shapes of the curves are, the more stable is the hearing instrument.

Test procedure

Figure 3.22 shows the exact course of the measuring for the basic frequency response.

a) Adjust the gain control to the reference test gain position i.e. with an input sound pressure level of 60 dB SPL. The gain should be adjusted so that the output sound pressure level at 1600 Hz is about 15 ± 1 dB lower than the OSPL 90 value at 1600 Hz.

b) The other controls should be set to positions that give the broadest frequency range.

c) Vary the frequency of the sound source over the recommended frequency range of 200 Hz to 8000 Hz keeping the input sound pressure level at 60 dB SPL.

d) Plot the ear simulator sound pressure level as a function of frequency.

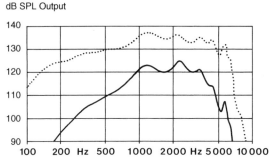

Figure 3.22: Basic frequency response

3.2.4 Battery current

The purpose of this test is to determine the current consumption of the hearing instrument in operation.

Test procedure

a) With the gain control in the reference test gain position, measure the battery current at the reference test frequency with an input sound pressure level of 60 dB SPL.

The direct-current measuring system must have the following characteristics:
1. An accuracy of ± 5% at the value of current measured.
2. A DC resistance not exceeding (50/I) Ω with the current being measured in mA.
3. An AC impedance not exceeding 1 Ω over the frequency range 20 Hz to 5000 Hz.

Note: One method of realizing Item 3 above is to bypass the current measuring instrument with an 8000 µF capacitor. However, the capacitor should not shunt the battery or the power supply.

3.2.5 Nonlinear distortions

The purpose of this test is to determine the degree of the amplitude nonlinearity in the sound output under specified conditions. The amplitude nonlinearity can be described in terms of:

a) Harmonic distortion
Harmonic distortion occurs when any part of the hearing instrument does not respond in proportion to the input signal. Harmonic distortion products are frequencies in the output of a hearing instrument which are integer multiples of the input frequency (fundamental). At high frequencies, the harmonic distortion products may fall outside the frequency range of the receiver. Therefore, nonlinearity is not sufficiently indicated by measurement of harmonic distortion at high frequencies. However, for the lower frequency range, the amount of harmonic distortion gives a reasonable indication of the hearing instrument's nonlinearity.

b) Intermodulation distortion
Intermodulation distortion occurs when the input is a signal composed of at least two frequencies. Such distortion products are frequencies in the output of the hearing instrument which are not in the input, but are sum and difference tones of the input frequencies. Determination of intermodulation distortion gives a better indication of nonlinearity in the high frequencies than measurement of harmonic distortion. Intermodulation distortion will not be addressed further here. In this section, the measurement of harmonic distortion will be discussed.

Harmonic distortion

Harmonic distortion is measured using a pure tone input signal having the frequency f. The frequencies of the harmonics are then nf, where n is an integer. Total harmonic distortion, or harmonic distortion of the nth order, is defined as the ratio of the output sound pressure of the harmonics to the output sound pressure of the total signal and will be expressed as a percentage. The total harmonic distortion is given by the formula:

$$k = \sqrt{\frac{P_2^2 + P_3^2 + P_4^2 + \ldots}{P_1^2 + P_2^2 + P_3^2 + P_4^2 + \ldots}}$$

and harmonic distortion of the nth order by the formula:

where p_1 is the sound pressure of the fundamental frequency of the signal in the ear simulator and p_2, p_3, p_4 ...p_n are the sound pressures of the second, third, fourth ...nth harmonics.

Test procedure

a) Adjust the gain control of the hearing instrument to the reference test gain position. The position of other controls must be reported; these should preferably be set to give the broadest bandwidth.

b) Vary the frequency of the sound source over the frequency range 200 Hz to 5000 Hz with an input sound pressure level of 70 dB and analyze the output signal for levels at the harmonic frequencies nf or record the total harmonic distortion content. The bandwidth of the filter should be stated. For continuous recording the sweep rate should be such that the response does not differ by more than 1 dB from the steady-state value at any frequency.
In the event that the response curve rises 12 dB or more from the SPL of the fundamental to that of the second harmonic for any test frequency, distortion tests at that frequency may be omitted.

c) Plot the harmonic distortion as a function of the frequency of the sound source and/or versus the input sound pressure level.

Figure 3.23 shows a harmonic distortion measurement in which the second and third harmonics are individually measured and plotted as a function of frequency (f). When, as in the example, the total harmonic distortion at a certain frequency also has been calculated, then the percentage of distortion for the individual harmonics can be obtained by applying the formula.

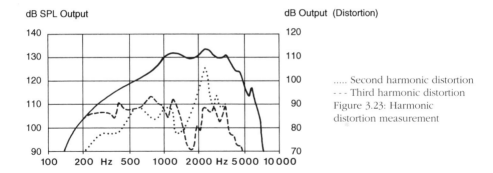

dB SPL Output   dB Output (Distortion)

..... Second harmonic distortion
- - - Third harmonic distortion
Figure 3.23: Harmonic
distortion measurement

a) How great is the harmonic distortion for the second harmonic component in %?
b) How great is the harmonic distortion for the third harmonic component in %?
c) How great is the total harmonic distortion in %?
As the distortion of a harmonic is equivalent to the factor of how much smaller
it is than the total harmonic distortion, then the harmonic distortion can be simply calculated.

a) Difference between the second harmonic and the total harmonic distortion:
   −34 dB
   $k_2 => -34\ dB \rightarrow 0.01995 = 2{,}0\%$

b) Difference between the third harmonic and the total harmonic distortion:
   −31 dB
   $k_3 => -31\ dB \rightarrow 0.0282 = 2{,}8\%$

c) In order to calculate the total harmonic distortion, the distortion of the individual harmonics must be quadratically added:

$$k_{Tot} = \sqrt{k_2^2 + k_3^2} = \sqrt{(0{,}0199)^2 + (0{,}0282)^2} = 0{,}0345 = 3{,}5\%$$

Figure 3.24 shows the harmonic distortion of an amplifier represented as a function of the input sound pressure level. When the harmonic distortion is plotted
in this manner, the frequency at which it was measured must be reported.

Distortion (%)

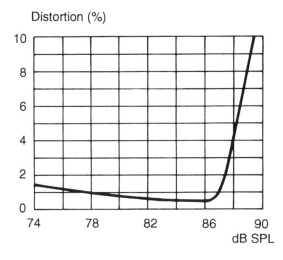

Figure 3.24: Harmonic distortion as a function of the input sound pressure level at 1000 Hz

3.2.6 Equivalent input noise level

Equivalent input noise level is a quantity which expresses the internally generated noise. It is imperative that the ambient noise in the test space be negligible when measuring equivalent input noise level.

Test procedure

a) Adjust the gain control of the hearing instrument to approximately the reference test position. A precise adjustment of the gain control is not strictly necessary. The position of the trimmers must be stated in the test report. Here again, the trimmers should be positioned so that the hearing instrument gives the broadest frequency response.

b) Measure the output sound pressure level L_S in the ear simulator at the reference test frequency with a pure tone input sound pressure level $L_1 = 60$ dB SPL.

Note: For hearing instruments with an automatic gain control (AGC), an input sound pressure level of 60 dB SPL may be too high and should be reduced to a level which ensures essentially linear input/output conditions. If this is the case, the input sound pressure level should be stated.

c) Switch off the sound source and measure the sound pressure level L_2 in the ear simulator. This is the internally generated noise. To ensure that the noise in the ear simulator and the ear simulator microphone system is adequately low, the measured noise should decrease by at least 10 dB when the hearing instrument is turned off.

d) Calculate the equivalent input noise level L_N as follows:

$$L_N = L_2 - (L_S - L_1)$$

where:
L_2 is the sound pressure level in the ear simulator as measured in Item c)
L_S is the sound pressure level in the ear simulator at the reference test frequency as measured in Item b)
L_1 is the input sound pressure level at the reference test frequency (generally 60 dB SPL)

Figure 3.25 is an equivalent input noise measurement curve for a hearing instrument which was measured in accordance with this procedure. (Above 8000 Hz, the noise level (L_2) of the hearing instrument can be read directly.)

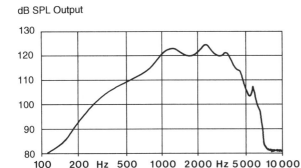

Figure 3.25: Equivalent input noise measurement of a hearing instrument

Example : $L_N = L_2 - (L_S - L_1) = 81dBSPL - (120dBSPL - 60dBSPL); L_N = 21dBSPL$

3.2.7 Induction coil measurement

To measure an induction coil in a hearing instrument, a current loop must be utilized which can supply a magnetic field of 10 mA/m. The magnetic field strength must remain constant within the frequency range of 100 Hz to 10 kHz. The field strength of 10 mA/m corresponds to an acoustic sound pressure level of 50 dB SPL. The gain control is adjusted to maximum when performing this measurement.

Instrumentation set-up

Figure 3.26 shows the set-up for measuring the induction coil of a hearing instrument.

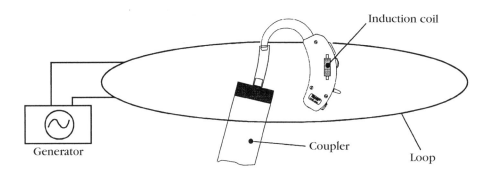

Figure 3.26: Induction coil measurement

The induction coil frequency response should be as close to the acoustic frequency response curve as possible. Some countries have standards which allow the induction coil frequency response to differ widely from the acoustic frequency response. In Scandinavian countries, where the use of the induction coil is widespread (through loop systems in nearly all public buildings), the standards for induction coil frequency response are quite strict. Switzerland, on the other hand, has no provisions concerning the deviation of the induction coil frequency response from the acoustic frequency response.

Figure 3.27 shows a comparison between the acoustic frequency response and the induction coil frequency response for a particular hearing instrument. It can be clearly seen that the induction coil is less sensitive at low frequencies compared to the microphone. The reason for this is to be found in the physics of inductivity. → The voltage which is induced in a coil is frequency dependent; that is, the higher the frequency, the higher is the induced voltage.

dB SPL Output

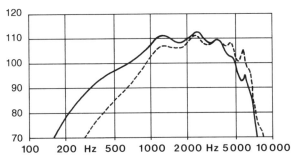

—— Acoustic amplification curve
---- Induction coil amplification
curve
Figure 3.27

3.2.8 Measuring of hearing instruments with automatic gain control (AGC) circuits

A standardized method of testing hearing instruments of any type with automatic gain control (AGC) circuits has been developed.
This includes devices which have compression and/or limiting properties with respect to the envelope of the input signal as well as devices which control the long-term average output level.

a) AGC is used to achieve compression. Put another way, the dynamic range of the output sound signal is reduced, the object being to preserve the integrity of the input waveform.

b) AGC circuits are often used for limiting gain instead of peak clipping (PC).

A limiting effect occurs when the shape of the input/output function flattens out at higher input levels. Output limitation is mainly used as a means of protecting the ear against excessively high output levels.

Explanation of terms

Automatic gain control (AGC)
A means by which the gain of a hearing instrument is automatically controlled as a function of the magnitude of the envelope of the input signal or other signal parameter.

Steady-state input/output graph
The graph illustrating the output sound pressure level as a function of the input sound pressure level for a specified frequency, both expressed in dB on identical linear scales. (Figure 3.28)

Lower AGC limit or AGC threshold
The input sound pressure level at which there is a reduction in the gain of 2 dB ± 0.5 dB with respect to linear gain. (Figure 3.28)

Compression ratio (between specified input sound pressure levels)
Under steady-state conditions, the ratio of the difference between two input sound pressure levels and the corresponding difference in the output sound pressure levels, both expressed in dB. (Figure 3.28)

Dynamic output characteristics
The output sound pressure envelope as a function of time when a pure tone input signal of a standard frequency and level is modulated by a square envelope pulse with a standard pulse amplitude. (Figure 3.29)

Attack time
The time interval between the abrupt increase in the input signal level and the point when the output sound pressure level from the hearing instrument with the AGC circuit stabilizes to within ± 2 dB of the elevated steady-state level. (Figure 3.29)

Attack time for the normal dynamic range of speech
The attack time when the initial input sound pressure level is 55 dB SPL and the increase in input sound pressure level is 25 dB.

Recovery time
The time interval between the abrupt reduction in the steady-state input signal level after the AGC amplifier has reached the steady-state output under elevated input conditions, and the point at which the output sound pressure level from the hearing instrument stabilizes again at within ± 2 dB of the lower steady-state level. (Figure 3.29)

Recovery time for the normal dynamic range of speech
The recovery time when the initial input sound pressure level is 80 dB SPL and the decrease in input sound pressure level is 25 dB.

Methods of measurements

Steady-state input/output graph

Graph showing the relationship between input sound pressure level and output sound pressure level. The gain control of the hearing instrument is adjusted to its maximum setting. A 1600 Hz pure tone input is delivered with a SPL of 40 dB and the output SPL measured. The output SPL is plotted on a graph as a function of the input SPL. The input sound pressure level is then increased in steps of 5 or 10 dB up to 100 dB SPL. At each step, the output SPL is measured and plotted on the graph. (Figure 3.28)

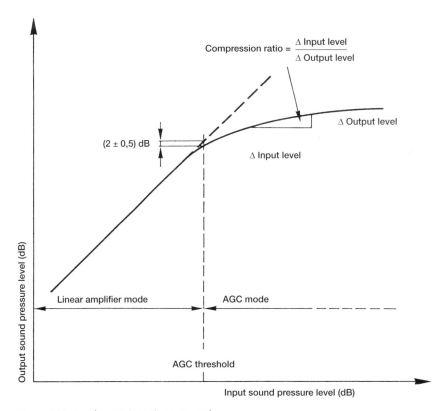

Figure 3.28: Steady-state input/output graph

Dynamic output characteristics (attack and release times)

The gain control is set full-on. A 1600 Hz (or 2500 Hz where appropriate) pure tone signal is delivered at 55 dB SPL. An adjustable gain control located after the AGC loop must be adjusted in such a manner that overload of the hearing instrument is avoided.
This signal is modulated by a square envelope pulse increasing the input level by 25 dB. The pulse length must be at least five times longer than the attack time being measured. If more than a single pulse is applied, the interval between two pulses must be at least five times the longest recovery time being measured.

Note: The loudspeaker employed for the measurement of dynamic output characteristics must be sufficiently free of transient distortion to ensure that any effect on test results is negligible. The output signal is monitored on a device such as an oscilloscope.

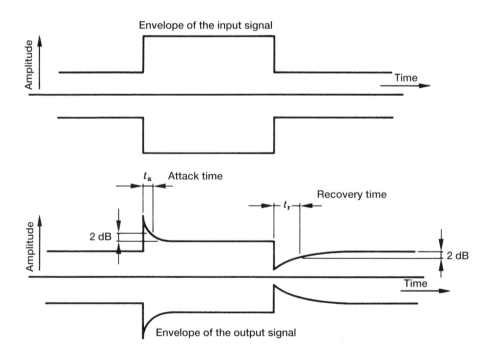

Figure 3.29: Dynamic output characteristic of a hearing instrument with AGC circuit

Example of an AGC measurement

a) Attack time at an abrupt increase from 55 to 80 dB SPL

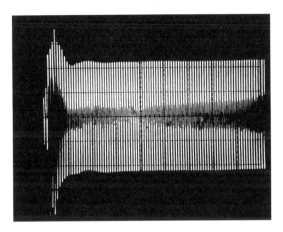

Figure 3.30: Measurement of the attack time (~5 ms) Scale: 5 ms/unit

b) Recovery time at an abrupt decrease from 80 to 55 dB SPL

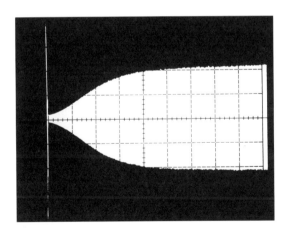

Figure 3.31: Measurement of the recovery time (~200 ms) Scale: 50 ms/unit

3.2.9 Measurement of hearing instruments with a directional microphone

In contrast to hearing instruments with omnidirectional microphones, for which the position of the hearing instrument in the measuring box does not play a major role, hearing instruments with a directional microphone require a special measuring arrangement.

1. In order to obtain valid results, hearing instruments with directional microphones must be measured in free field. If testing is performed in too small a chamber (e.g. in a normal sound box) then false results are obtained in the low frequencies (< 500 Hz). Figure 3.32 illustrates false results in the low frequencies when the sound box is too small.

dB SPL Output

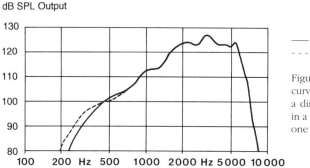

—— False measurement (small box)
- - - Correct measurement (large box)

Figure 3.32: Frequency response curves for a hearing instrument with a directional microphone obtained in a sound box that is too small and one that is large enough.

2. The front and rear microphone ports must lie on the loudspeaker axis. The axis of the control microphone (using the comparison method) must lie in the reference plane (See Figure 3.33).

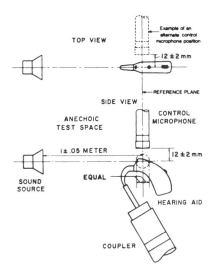

Figure 3.33: Configuration for measuring a hearing instrument with directional microphone in accordance with ANSI Standard [1]

Figure 3.34 shows a correct arrangement for a hearing instrument with a directional microphone in a sound box with the sound source (loudspeaker) in the box cover. If a sound box has a loudspeaker beneath the test plane then the instrument must be turned 180°.

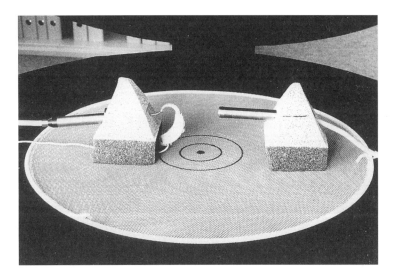

Figure 3.34: Measuring arrangement for a hearing instrument with a directional microphone

3. If a hearing instrument with a directional microphone is incorrectly arranged in the sound box (e.g. not facing the sound source) then a damping of the measured signal will occur. The measured gain of the hearing instrument will be lower than the actual value.

dB SPL Output

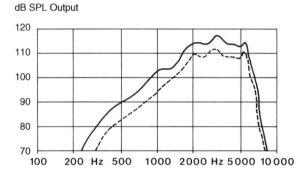

—— 0° incidence (from the front)
- - - 90° incidence (from the side)
Figure 3.35: Frequency response curves measured with correct (0°) and incorrect (90°) arrangement of a hearing instrument with a directional microphone (Directional characteristic: cardioid)

It is interesting to observe the directional characteristics of a hearing instrument with a directional microphone. To do this, the instrument is placed directly in front of the sound source (0°) for the first measurement while for the second measurement, the sound comes from directly behind the unit. Figure 3.36 shows such a measurement of a microphone with a cardioid characteristic.

dB SPL Output

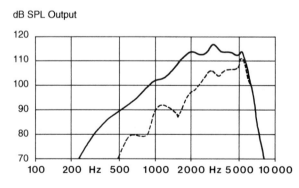

—— 0° incidence (from the front)
- - - 180° incidence (from behind)
Figure 3.36: Hearing instrument comparison measurement in free field with 0° incidence (sound from the front) compared with 180° (sound from behind).

3.3 Measuring on KEMAR

When hearing instruments are measured in a sound box then the measured values (e.g. for quality control) are comparable. However, since such measurements differ from those made in actual ears, they are of little value in assessing the performance of the hearing instrument in use. This is especially true when attempting to compare hearing instruments of different construction. The results measured in a sound box provide no information regarding the type of hearing instrument (behind-the-ear unit → microphone above the ear/in-the-ear → microphone in the ear), nor the effect of shadowing of the sound by the head and body. Neither is the effect of the ear canal resonance taken into account when testing is carried out in a coupler (or ear simulator).

An anthropometric mannequin has been developed that makes possible accurate and reproducible measurements which are representative of results obtained from real ears. This mannequin has proved especially useful in the designing of hearing instruments. The mannequin is constructed with two pinnas fabricated of a flexible plastic and two ear simulators located at the ends of tubes representing median ear canals. In addition, the mannequin has a torso and arms extending to the waist, which enables inclusion of sound diffraction around the body when measuring. This mannequin was developed by Knowles Electronics and is called KEMAR (Knowles Electronics Manikin for Acoustical Research). The head and torso dimensions of KEMAR are based on the average size of more than 4000 men. The median values used for construction of the pinnas and ear canals were derived from a study of 12 men and women.

Figure 3.37 shows KEMAR's head and part of its torso. KEMAR is mounted on a turntable which is used when meausuring polar responses. In the bottom photograph, the placement of the B&K ear simulator can be seen inside KEMAR's head. To allow flexibility for research purposes, the pinnas can be changed (e.g. replaced by smaller ones) and the head turned with respect to the body.

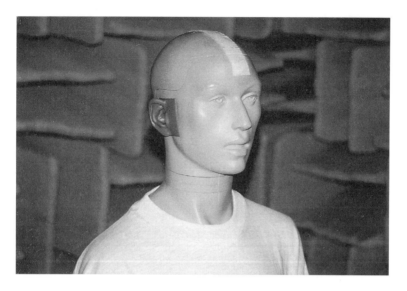

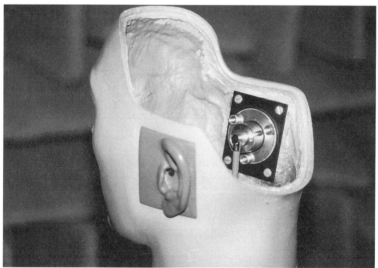

Figure 3.37: KEMAR body mannequin

3.3.1 The ear canal resonance of KEMAR

Figure 3.38 shows the open ear canal resonance of KEMAR. There is a distinct resonance of about 17 dB at 2.5 kHz. In order to measure this open ear canal resonance, KEMAR is placed in a free field and the sound pressure at the ear drum is measured via the ear simulator.

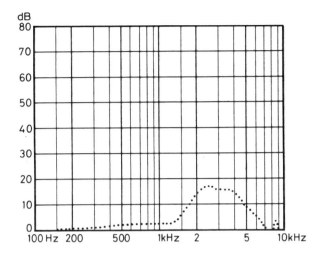

Figure 3.38: Open ear canal resonance of KEMAR

3.3.2 In-situ measuring and insertion gain

With a BTE or an ITE hearing instrument fitted on KEMAR, it is possible to measure the SPL produced by the instrument at the end of the ear canal via the ear simulator. This measurement is called in-situ gain.

The ear canal resonance is lost by occluding the ear canal with an earmold or in-the-ear hearing instrument. The hearing instrument must compensate for this loss. In other words, showing the effective gain of the hearing instrument requires that the open ear canal resonance be subtracted from the in-situ gain. This 'effective amplification' is called insertion gain.

These definitions are applicable not only to KEMAR measurements but also to hearing instrument fitting.

In-situ gain – open ear canal resonance = insertion gain

Figure 3.39 shows the three curves for a hearing instrument measurement on KEMAR. The measurements are made with an in-the-ear hearing instrument.

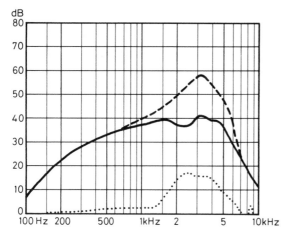

- - - In-situ measurement
······ Open ear canal resonance
—— Insertion gain (Difference
between curve - - - and ······)
Figure 3.39: Insertion gain as measured on KEMAR

3.3.3 Measurement of a polar response

With KEMAR on a turntable, it is possible to determine the directional characteristics of a hearing instrument.

It is also possible to measure the influence of the head (head shadow) on a hearing instrument with an omnidirectional microphone.

Measurement procedure

With the hearing instrument in place on KEMAR, a pure tone signal (e.g. 500 Hz, 1000 Hz or 2000 Hz) is presented, initially at 0° incidence. As KEMAR is turned once around its own axis, the sound pressure (amplification) is recorded as a function of the angle of rotation. Such a curve is called a polar response.

Figure 3.40 shows a diagram of a polar response of KEMAR without a hearing instrument. The influence of the head and pinnas at different frequencies and from different directions can be observed.

Note: High frequencies are affected more strongly by sound diffraction around the head than low frequencies.

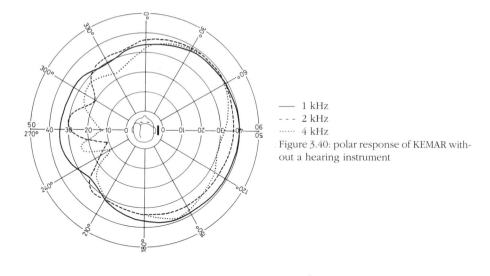

— 1 kHz
- - - 2 kHz
······ 4 kHz

Figure 3.40: polar response of KEMAR without a hearing instrument

Figure 3.41 shows a polar response with a behind-the-ear unit with a directional microphone. We can see that sound coming from behind is attenuated by up to 20 dB. The main effect (suppression of noise) of hearing instruments with a directional microphone is the damping of sound from behind.

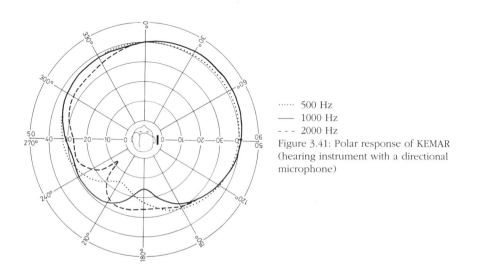

······ 500 Hz
— 1000 Hz
- - - 2000 Hz

Figure 3.41: Polar response of KEMAR (hearing instrument with a directional microphone)

3.4 Measurement standards

Standards have been established which delineate the properties of hearing instruments to be reported, and specify how these properties are to be determined and described.

Hearing instrument manufacturers would like to describe their products as comprehensively as possible. The hearing healthcare professional, on the other hand, would prefer a standard description simple enough not to require reference to the standard publication in order to interpret it. In addition, the standard measuring methods should be as practical, simple and reproducible as possible.

3.4.1 IEC Standard (1983) → see section [3.2]

The electroacoustic characteristics of hearing instruments to be reported according to the IEC Standard (1983) have been thoroughly covered in section [3.2] and will not be addressed further in this chapter.

3.4.2 ANSI Standard (1987)[1]

This standard has been developed under the American National Standards Institude (ANSI) Standards Committee method of procedure under sponsorship of the Acoustical Society of America (ASA). The ANSI Standard and the IEC Standard are the most important standards and are widely used today. The ANSI Standard is used in Australia and America as well as several other countries.

Measurements in accordance with the ANSI Standard are made with a 2 cc coupler.

In this section, ANSI's terminology will be briefly explained. All measurements in the examples are made with a PHONAK, PICONET 231X. (Try to carry out these measurements in your sound box!)

Saturation sound pressure level for 90 dB input sound pressure level (SSPL 90)
With the gain control of the hearing instrument full-on and an input sound pressure of 90 dB SPL, the output sound pressure is determined from 200 to 5000 Hz. → Figure 3.42.

dB SPL Output

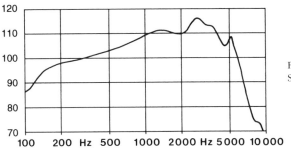

Figure 3.42: Measurement of the SSPL 90 curve

HF-average SSPL 90
The maximum output sound pressure level with full-on gain at 3 frequencies (1000/1600/2500 Hz) are added and the sum divided by 3. The sound pressure level so obtained is called the HF-average SSPL 90. HF-average SSPL 90 from the curve in Figure 3.42: 112 dB SPL.

Full-on gain
With the gain control of the hearing instrument set at full-on and an input sound pressure of 60 dB SPL, full-on gain is recorded as a function of frequency. If a 60 dB input SPL would overload the hearing instrument, then an input of 50 dB SPL is used (Figure 3.43).

dB Gain

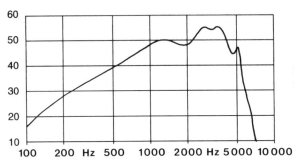

Figure 3.43 : Full-on gain curve measurement

HF-Average full-on gain
The average of the full-on gain at the frequencies 1000/1600/2500 Hz. HF-average full-on gain from the curve in Figure 3.43: 50 dB.

Reference test position
With an input sound pressure of 60 dB SPL, the amplification control is adjusted so that the average (1000/1600/2500 Hz) of the output sound pressure level is 17 dB lower than the HF-average SSPL 90. Reference test position from the curve Figure 3.44: 95 dB SPL.

Reference test gain
The average of the gain of a 60 dB SPL input at 1000/1600/2500 Hz with the gain control set at the reference test position. Reference test gain from the curve Figure 3.44: 35 dB.

ASA-frequency range
A frequency response curve is obtained with the gain control in the reference test position and the average output SPL of 1000/1600/2500 Hz is determined. A horizontal line is drawn on the graph 20 dB below this average value. The points at which the line intersects the frequency response curve indicate the ASA-frequency range.
ASA-frequency range from the curve in Figure 3.44: 230 Hz–6000 Hz.

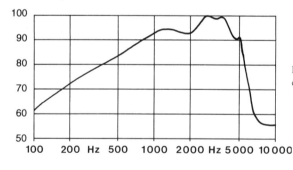

Figure 3.44: Frequency response curve with reference test gain

Induction coil sensitivity
The hearing instrument is set to the "T" (telephone input) mode and placed in a sinusoidal alternating magnetic field having an rms magnetic field strength of 10 mA/m at 1000 Hz. The gain control is set to full-on and the hearing instrument is oriented to produce the greatest coupler sound pressure level.
Induction coil sensitivity at 1000 Hz as shown in Figure 3.45: 97 dB SPL.

dB SPL Output

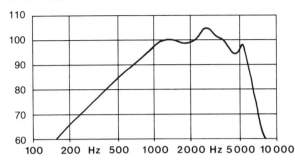

Figure 3.45: Frequency response curve of the induction coil sensitivity

Battery current
The battery current is determined with the hearing instrument adjusted to the reference test position. The battery current is measured at this position with an input sound pressure level of 65 dB SPL/1000 Hz. Battery current of the unit: 1.55 mA.

Equivalent input noise level
The equivalent input noise level L_n is measured with the gain control in the reference test position. It is calculated as follows:
L_{av} = average dB SPL output at 1000/1600/2500 Hz
L_2 = noise level of the unit in the reference test position
L_n = $L_2 - (L_{av} - 60)$ dB SPL
Equivalent input noise level from the curve in Figure 3.44: 21 dB SPL.

Harmonic distortion
The gain control is adjusted to the reference test position and the input sound pressure level increased to 70 dB SPL. The harmonic distortion is measured at 500, 800 and 1600 Hz. In the event the specified frequency response curve rises 12 dB or more between any distortion test frequency and its second harmonic, distortion tests at that frequency may be omitted.
Total harmonic distortion at 500 Hz: < 2%.
Total harmonic distortion at 800 Hz: < 2%.
Total harmonic distortion at 1600 Hz: < 1%.

dB SPL Output   dB Output (Distortion)

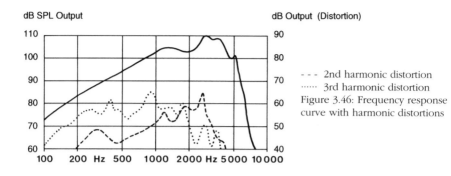

- - - 2nd harmonic distortion

······ 3rd harmonic distortion

Figure 3.46: Frequency response curve with harmonic distortions

4 Hearing instrument transducer

One of the most important components in the hearing instrument are its electroacoustic transducers.

Each hearing instrument has a microphone which picks up the acoustic signal and converts it into an electrical signal. The hearing instrument amplifier then modifies this signal according to hearing loss configuration and feeds it to the receiver. The receiver converts the electrical signal again into a sound signal appropriate for the hearing-impaired user.

There are a wide variety of electroacoustic transducers on the market. The different types may be characterized primarily in terms of:
– Technology
– Size
– Quality
– Price.

The correct choice of electroacoustic transducer is tantamount to an optimal acoustic fitting. Therefore, the different types of transducers will be discussed in detail.

4.1 The microphone

Following World War II, a number of research projects were undertaken with the purpose of determining a communications frequency band which would allow optimal understanding of speech under various conditions. These studies showed that, under favorable conditions, a frequency band of 300 Hz to 3000 Hz was most suitable for people with normal hearing.

Under worse conditions where loudness, noise, and distortion interfered with listening tasks, this band (300 Hz to 3000 Hz) still gave the best speech understanding (i.e. better than a narrower or broader frequency band).

This research had a strong influence on the entire field of telecommunications. Telephones today still have a frequency band of around 400 Hz to 5000 Hz.

dB SPL Output

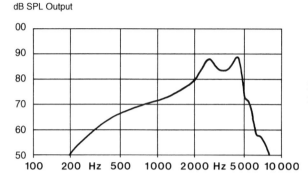

Figure 4.1: Transmission of a modern telephone (Tritel, 1990)

The optimal frequency band for speech understanding via a hearing instrument has also been the focus of much post-World War II research.

In these studies, speech comprehensibility tests with and without background noise were given to hearing-impaired subjects. Results indicated that a frequency band which was either flat or increasing at 6 dB/octave between 300 Hz and 4000 Hz (the frequency band is sharply cut above and below this range) was best for speech understanding for nearly all the hearing-impaired subjects.

An electroacoustic transducer with approximately this frequency pass band available at that time was the electromagnetic microphone.

dB

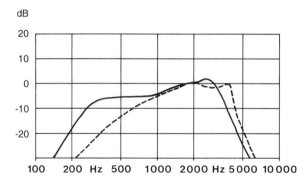

Figure 4.2: Frequency response curve of electromagnetic microphones

In the mid-sixties, increasingly greater demands were made of hearing instruments which could no longer be satisfied by the electromagnetic microphone. For one thing a broader and flatter frequency response was desired (so that one could fully enjoy the music of the Beatles). More and more people with slight hearing impairments were being fitted. For them things such as enjoyment of music and natural sounds as well as recognition of voices were important.

In the late sixties, a microphone with a broader and flatter frequency response became practical for hearing instrument application due to technological developments. This was the piezo-electric ceramic microphone.

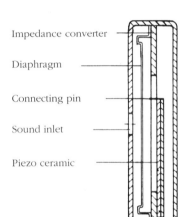

Impedance converter

Diaphragm

Connecting pin

Sound inlet

Piezo ceramic

Figure 4.3: Construction of a ceramic microphone

Figure 4.3 shows the construction of a ceramic microphone. It contains a flexible element made out of two strips of a piezo ceramic bonded together. Sound pressure variations move the diaphragm. These movements are then mechanically transmitted to the piezo ceramic via the connecting pin. When this piezo ceramic moves in phase with the sound, an alternating voltage is produced (again in phase with the sound). This element is extremely sensitive to electrostatic interference because of its exceptionally high impedance. Therefore an electrical impedance converter (amplifier) is necessary and is positioned directly adjacent to the element in the microphone housing. This element converts the electrical impedance so that there is a relatively low-resistance output at the external microphone terminals.
The power required for the microphone is drawn from the hearing instrument into which the microphone is built.
Such an impedance converter contains a field effect transistor. Figure 4.4 shows the frequency responses of a ceramic and a magnetic microphone.

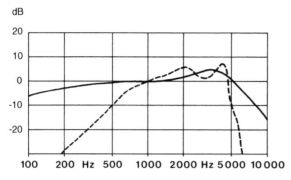

— Ceramic microphone
- - - Magnetic microphone
Figure 4.4: Frequency response of
a ceramic and a magnetic microphone [9]

The ceramic microphone has in fact a broader frequency response than the magnetic microphone (of the same size). Yet, despite its superiority to the magnetic microphone, the ceramic microphone has become obsolete in hearing instrument production. The reason for this?

The main problem with the ceramic microphone was its high sensitivity to vibrations at low frequencies (e.g. mechanical feedback, friction noise). This led
the microphone manufacturers to look for other, low vibration systems and, at
the beginning of the seventies, it became possible to produce an even better
microphone suitable for use in hearing instruments.
This was the electret-condenser microphone. The electret-condenser microphone works according to the electrostatic transducer principle. Condenser microphones consist of a thin metal diaphragm and a rigid metal backplate making up
the electrodes of an air dielectric capacitor. A DC voltage (polarization voltage)
is applied across the two electrodes. The effect of sound pressure on the
diaphragm is a variation of capacitance in accordance with the sound pressure
variations. This variation in capacitance is, in turn, transformed into voltage
variations. An AC voltage appears over a high ohmic resistor (being part of the
polarization circuit) and represents an analog of the sound picked up.

The DC voltage required for normal condenser microphones is not needed for
electret microphones, which possess a permanent electrical field and are comparable to permanent magnets.

The "electret" element is manufactured from high-insulation plastics such as
Teflon, in which a permanent electrostatic charge has been set up through
special processes.

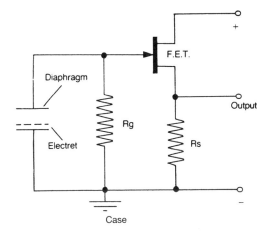

Figure 4.5: Electret condenser microphone circuit with an impedance converter (Knowles [12])

The electret condenser microphone has as high a resistance as the ceramic microphone. Therefore, the electret microphone also requires an impedance converter (field effect transistor) which is built into the microphone capsule. It is because of this impedance converter that a current supply is required for the electret condenser microphone.

Now we should consider sensitivity to vibrations. The heavier the diaphragm, the more sensitive it is to vibrations. As the diaphagm (film) is extremely light in the case of an electret condenser microphone, it is much less sensitive to vibrations than ceramic microphones.

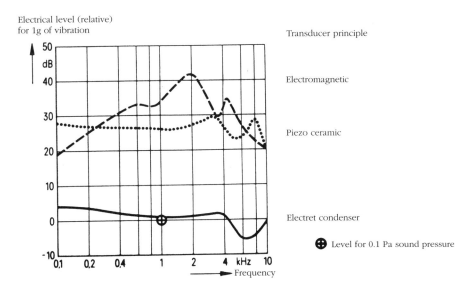

Figure 4.6: Sensitivity to vibration of different types of microphones (Knowles [10])

Figure 4.7 shows the frequency response of two electret condenser microphones. It is possible to maintain an extended linear frequency response (100 Hz to 15 kHz). A microphone with a resonance of 4 kHz is frequently used in hearing instrument applications.

This resonance can be reduced in frequency to around 2.5 to 3 kHz by using a sound tube to the microphone (extension of the microphone in the hearing instrument housing). The intent is to compensate for the loss in acoustical amplification (ear canal resonance) due to occlusion of the ear canal with closed earmolds.

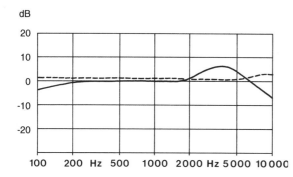

Figure 4.7: Possible frequency response curves for electret condenser microphones

4.1.1 The omnidirectional microphone (pressure sensor)

The omnidirectional microphone is a pressure sensor in that the diaphragm is moved exclusively by the sound pressure. When the pressure sensor is located in a sound field, the diaphragm movement depends only on sound pressure variations regardless of which direction the sound is coming from. A pressure sensor is in fact a microphone with a spherical pick-up characteristic.

Figure 4.8 shows a longitudinal section of an omnidirectional microphone. The omnidirectional microphone has one sound port and the sound is directed at one side of the diaphragm.

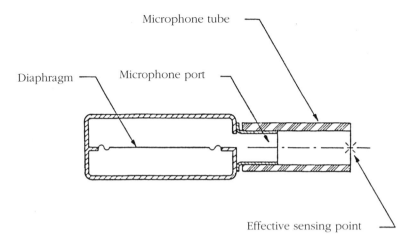

Microphone tube

Diaphragm

Microphone port

Effective sensing point

Figure 4.8: Section of an omnidirectional microphone

The directional characteristic of a microphone is shown by a polar plot. The sound source is moved in a circle around the microphone, and the microphone's output is plotted relative to that at 0° incidence. Figure 4.9 shows the polar response for an omnidirectional microphone. The solid circular line represents the directional characteristic in a free field. → The omnidirectional microphone has a spherical characteristic in that sound emanating from all directions is picked up with equal strength.

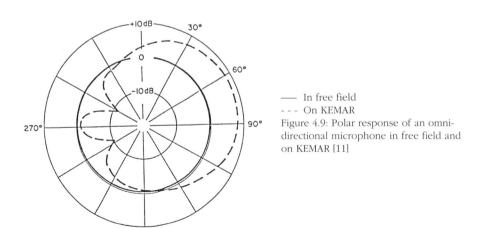

—— In free field
- - - On KEMAR
Figure 4.9: Polar response of an omnidirectional microphone in free field and on KEMAR [11]

The dashed curve represents the KEMAR response for the omnidirectional microphone and demonstrates clearly the influence of the head (head shadow, reflections).

Advantages and disadvantages of the omnidirectional microphone

+ Small
+ Full sonority, good low frequency transmission
+ Good vibrational damping
+ Low noise
− Spherical characteristic is problematic in background noise

4.1.2 The directional microphone (pressure gradient sensor)

Directional microphones have two sound ports such that sound is also directed to the rear side of the diaphragm. By careful dimensioning of the sound paths, different directional characteristics can be produced. The directional microphone reacts better to sound emanating from a certain direction.

Figure 4.10 shows a section of a directional microphone. The two sound ports lead to a small cavity which is divided into two chambers by the diaphragm. This diaphragm only determines the difference in air pressure between the two sides and transduces this into an electrical output signal. When the air pressure in both chambers is of equal level and phase, there is no net effect of pressure on the diaphragm and thus, no electrical output signal.
In order to prevent sound coming from behind reaching the diaphragm first, there is a time delay acoustical network (fine filter, mesh) connected to the rear port so that the sound reaches both sides of the diaphragm simultaneously. Thus, the pressure on both sides of the diaphragm will be equal and there will be no movement of the diaphragm (i.e. no electrical signal).

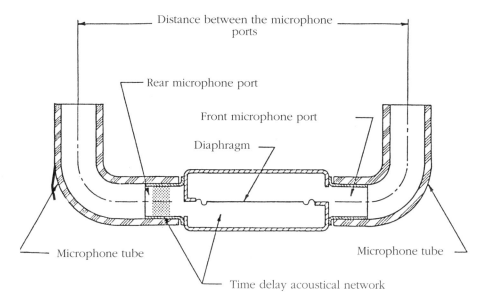

Figure 4.10: Longitudinal section of a directional microphone [11]

A directional microphone tested in free field typically shows a cardioid polar pattern, as illustrated by the solid curve in Figure 4.11. However, the directional characteristic of the microphone is quite different when the head shadow effect is taken into account (dashed curve).

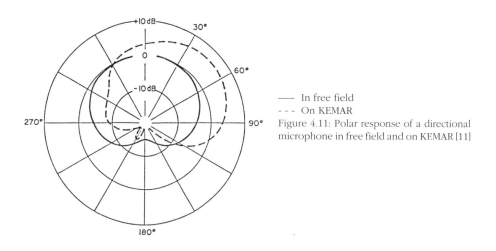

—— In free field
- - - On KEMAR
Figure 4.11: Polar response of a directional microphone in free field and on KEMAR [11]

The effective polar sensitivity of the directional microphone depends on how it is built into the hearing instrument. This is influenced by a number of factors including arrangement of the microphone ports and their distance from one another, the dimensions of the delay tube and the time delay acoustical network, and even the shape of the hearing instrument housing.

Therefore it is possible for the same directional microphone to exhibit different polar pickup characteristics. Figure 4.12 shows the difference in directionality that can result from changes in a single parameter.

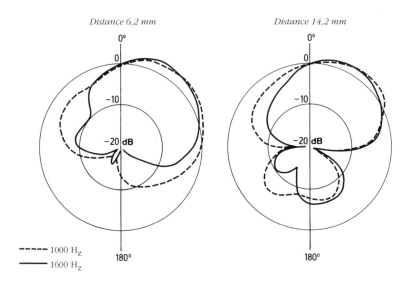

Figure 4.12: Polar sensitivity at different distances of the microphone ports [13]

As has already been shown in Chapter [3.2.9], (Measurement of hearing instruments with a directional microphone), the directional microphone has a frequency response with greater amplitude in the high frequencies than does the omnidirectional microphone.

Combined with the directionality of the directional microphone, this results in a notable improvement in speech intelligibility in a noisy environment.

If the rear port in a directional microphone is closed it then exhibits a spherical characteristic and flat frequency response. (Figure 4.13)

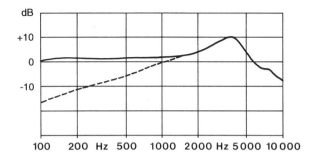

— Rear port closed
- - - Rear port open
Figure 4.13: Frequency response of a directional microphone with open and closed rear port

In certain hearing instruments, the hearing healthcare professional can close the rear microphone port by means of a slide, thereby making it effectively a hearing instrument without a directional microphone. (Tip: when possible, fit the hearing instrument with the directional microphone operative (slide open); the hearing-impaired wearer will likely be pleased with the effect).

Closing of the rear inlet is only possible, however, for hearing instruments with an amplification < 60 dB (2 cc coupler); at greater levels of amplification internal feedback (whistling) results from closing the rear port.

Another reason that few powerful hearing instruments utilize a directional microphone is that directional microphones are more sensitive to vibration than omnidirectional microphones. That is, the vibration damping of a directional microphone in a hearing instrument requires considerably more space than an omnidirectional microphone. Today, hearing instruments with directional microphones are seldom fitted despite the advantages in noisy surroundings.

The main reasons for this are:

1. Many hearing instrument manufacturers offer units with directional microphones only as an option.

2. Powerful hearing instruments with directional microphones are rare.

3. The hearing healthcare professional is not sufficiently aware of the enormous advantages of directional microphones.

Advantages and disadvantages of directional microphones

+ As yet, the most effective method for improving speech intelligibility in noisy environments.

– Poorer vibration damping than omnidirectional microphones.

– Directional effect is not desirable in all listening situations (e.g. music).

4.1.3 Special microphones

In sections [4.1.1] and [4.1.2], two types of microphones which differ in their directional characteristics are discussed. In this section, another microphone which differs in its amplitude response will be touched on: the slope microphone. This microphone is an omnidirectional microphone. The amplitude response of the slope microphone differs primarily in the low frequency range. Compare the flat frequency response of an omnidirectional microphone as shown in Figure 4.7 on Page 68 with the 4 different slope microphone frequency responses in Figure 4.14. One can clearly see the fall in sensitivity in the lower frequencies.

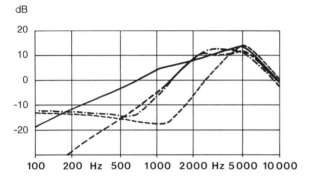

Figure 4.14: Various slope microphones [12]

Slope microphones are used principally in small in-the-ear units. Slope microphones also allow the elimination of a sophisticated filter circuit from the hearing instrument. The main disadvantage of slope microphones is their relatively poor signal-to-noise ratio at low frequencies.

4.1.4 Summary

The electret condenser microphones used in hearing instruments today are of a superior quality. They exhibit a (desirable) flat frequency response to well above 10 kHz and an equivalent input noise level of 23 dB SPL (A-weighted). (The A-filter approximates the sensitivity of human hearing, i.e., low (f<500 Hz) and high (f>5000 Hz) frequency components are less emphasised than frequencies in the intermediate band in which the human ear is most sensitive). This 23 dB SPL equivalent input noise level is almost always the dominant noise source in the hearing instrument and it is interesting to consider this in relation to ambient noise. Consider the following table in which natural ambient noises are compared.

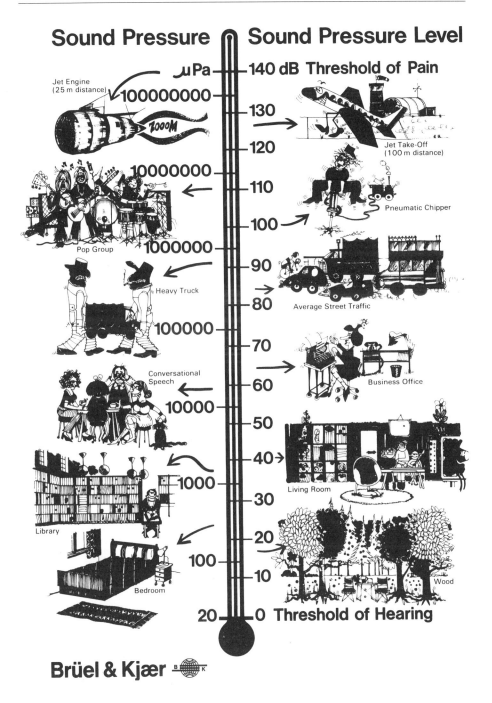

Figure 4.15: Various ambient noises

It can be seen (Figure 4.15) that the microphone noise (23 dB SPL) is far below the level of most natural ambient noises and thus cannot be detected in their presence.

The current consumption of an electret condenser microphone in a hearing instrument is 50 μA maximum (typically 30 μA). This means (how often this is misunderstood) that the microphone current consumption in relation to that of the hearing instrument as a whole is neglible.

Future

Various research institutes are working on the next generation of microphones → the silicon microphone. It will be produced in a manner similar to that for an integrated circuit. The advantages of a silicon microphone are 'simple' mechanical production and tighter sensitivity tolerances. The disadvantage is that as yet there is still too much noise. The target of a new silicon microphone design will be a much smaller microphone with the same performance as an electret microphone.

4.2 Hearing instrument receivers

The function of the hearing instrument receiver is to convert the amplified electrical signal into an acoustic signal again. The hearing instrument's receiver must be highly effective, capable of producing as great an output SPL as possible.

The hearing instrument receiver works in accordance with the electromagnetic principle.

A current flowing through a coil causes it to behave like a magnet. That is, it forms a magnetic north and south pole depending on the direction of the current. An alternating current flowing through the coil causes a shift in polarity of the coil corresponding to the alternating current and thus, a continual change in the direction of the magnetic field lines. An alternating magnetic field is the result. Figure 4.16 shows a section of a hearing instrument receiver with the main parts identified.

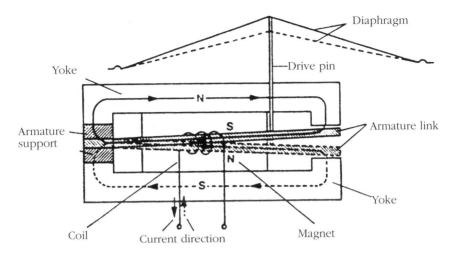

Figure 4.16: Electromagnetic hearing instrument receiver

The armature of the receiver is a thin, magnetically permeable metal reed with a coil of fine wire around it. When the receiver is not in operation, the armature rests between the two yokes of the magnetic system. When current flows through the coil, a north or south pole is produced at the free-moving end of the armature according to the direction of the current. The armature is thus alternately attracted to or repelled from the permanent magnets.

In other words, an alternating current flowing through the coil results in deflections of the armature to either side corresponding to the change of direction of the current. The armature acts on the diaphragm via the drive pin causing the development of sound pressure variations in the adjacent volume of air.

Various resonances are present in an electromagnetic sound transducer:
– Electrical resonance: Coil and own capacitance.
– Mechanical resonance: Diaphragm size and material.
– Acoustic resonance: receiver volume, tube length and diameter, residual ear cavity.

These resonances together shape the frequency response which also varies dependant on external factors. Particularly in the case of behind-the-ear units, the hook of the hearing instrument and the sound bore in the earmold affect the acoustic resonances. Lengthening of the receiver tube or reduction of its diameter causes the resonances of the receiver frequency curve to be displaced towards the lower frequencies and vice versa (see Chapter 5).

4.2.1 The Class A receiver

In section 4.2, the basic properties of an electromagnetic receiver were described. In the three following sections (4.2.1 to 4.2.3), electromagnetic receivers will be considered together with a given amplifier (output stage). The name of the receiver is determined by the type of output amplifier employed.

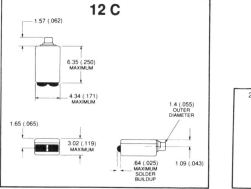
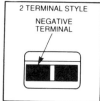

Figure 4.17: Class A receiver (Knowles, Datasheet [12])

Thus Class A receivers are connected to Class A output amplifiers.

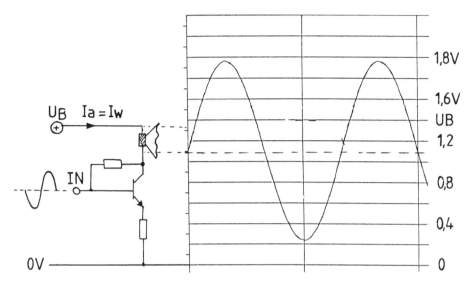

Figure 4.18: Circuit diagram of an output amplifier with Class A receiver

The Class A receiver has two terminals. The operating current (I_A) flows through the receiver and produces a magnetic field. The reed of the receiver is deflected under the influence of this magnetic field. To counteract this deflection, the reed is mechanically linked to the other side by the transducer manufacturer. As soon as the operating current for the receiver begins to flow, the reed moves to the middle position and can then swing freely.

Important: It is for this reason that the Class A receiver must be correctly polarized i.e. the receiver wires must not be reversed.

Note

As shown in Figure 4.18, the operating point of the hearing instrument receiver is close to the battery voltage. Therefore it is possible to have a deflection from 1.1 V. The amplifier cannot cause a deflection above the battery voltage (U_B). The high inductivity of the receiver (= coil) enables the energy to be stored in the coil. This energy is released when the supply voltage is exceeded. → Result: about 2.2 V maximum alternating voltage over the receiver.

Advantages and disadvantages of Class A receivers

+ As long as the receiver does not exceed its limits, there is little distortion.
+ Better than other receiver solutions.
− Class A receivers with a final stage have a fixed operating current which is relatively high.

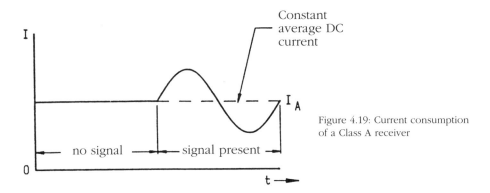

Figure 4.19: Current consumption of a Class A receiver

4.2.2 The Class B receiver (push-pull receiver)

In contrast to the Class A receiver, the push-pull receiver has three terminals.

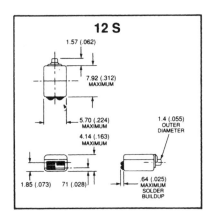
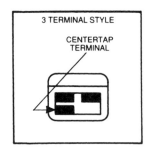

Figure 4.20: Push-pull receiver (Knowles, Datasheet [12])

The push-pull receiver has a coil with a center tap. This center tap is connected to the supply voltage U_B which results, in fact, in two Class A receivers. Both halves of the receiver now receive equal signals but out of phase by 180°.

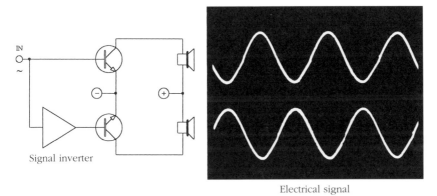

Electrical signal

Figure 4.21: Operation of a push-pull amplifier/receiver (1)

As the receiver again inverts the two signals through its winding with the center tap the resultant effect (deflection of the diaphragm), is an addition of the two signals.

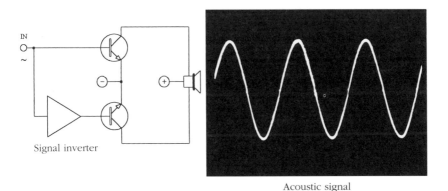

Acoustic signal

Figure 4.22: Operation of a push-pull amplifier/receiver (2)

The result is a maximum acoustic amplitude which is about twice that of a Class A receiver's output.

Current consumption

A further advantage of Class B receivers over Class A receivers is that the Class B amplifier consumes current dependent on the output signal. That is, the smaller the electrical signal at the receiver, the smaller is the current consumption. If no signal is present, then only a very small quiescent current flows.

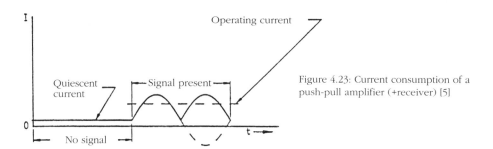

Figure 4.23: Current consumption of a push-pull amplifier (+receiver) [5]

As the reed of the receiver is only deflected by the signal from the central position (only a small quiescent current is flowing), the push-pull receiver has no definite polarity; that is, the two signal inputs of the push-pull receiver can be reversed.

→ Note: The reversal of the receiver terminals inverts the acoustic output signal (acoustic signal and magnetic field are phase displaced by 180°). This can cause acoustic or induction coil problems (feedback!), especially in the case of powerful behind-the-ear units.

Advantages and disadvantages of push-pull receivers

+ Higher maximum output sound pressure possible (6 dB higher than with Class A).
+ Negligible quiescent current and high current consumption only when necessary.
− The method of operation of the Class B amplifier results in cross-over distortions when the signal passes through zero. The distortion varies inversely with the quiescent current.

4.2.3 The Class D receiver

A Class D receiver is an electromagnetic receiver with an integrated Class D amplifier; that is, the output amplifier (here Class D) is built into the housing of the receiver. The Class D receiver has 3 terminals which are:

1. + battery positive
2. – battery negative   Current supply for the Class D amplifier
3. ~ input signal

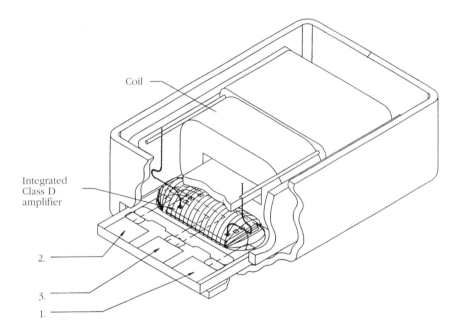

Figure 4.24: Class D receiver (Knowles [5])

How does a Class D amplifier work?

The Class D amplifier (also called a switching amplifier) converts the analog input signal into a digital signal.

More precisely: A pulse-width modulated signal (PWM) is produced from the analog signal by means of a square wave generator and a comparator. The sampling frequency is at about 100 kHz. (See Figure 4.25)

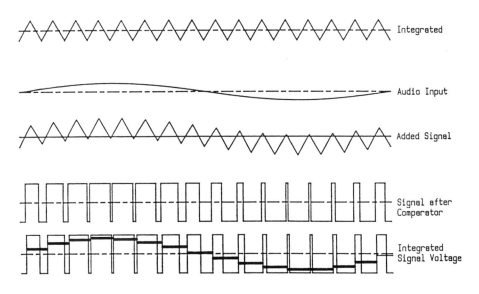

Integrated

Audio Input

Added Signal

Signal after
Comparator

Integrated
Signal Voltage

Figure 4.25: Curve shapes of a Class D amplifier in a Knowles Class D receiver [5]

The pulse width modulated square wave signal controls a power switch which alternately charges the coil of the receiver with a positive and negative supply voltage.

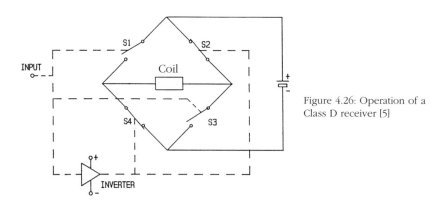

Figure 4.26: Operation of a Class D receiver [5]

As the receiver coil cannot transfer the high sampling frequency (100 kHz), an analog signal is again produced from the pulse width modulated square wave signal.

Current consumption

The main advantage of the Class D receiver is its low current consumption! Although the quiescent current is more or less equivalent to that of the Class B receiver, the operating current of the Class D receiver is 20 to 40% lower.

Advantages and disadvantages of a Class D receiver

+ Current consumption
+ Reduced size (by integration of the output stage into the receiver housing)
+ Good acoustic properties as long as the receiver is not operated at its performance limits (maximum sound pressure)
− Cost (particularly for in-the-ear units where the receiver is often invaded by debris)
− Today's Class D receivers are suitable for high power hearing instruments. However, this is not yet possible. Reason: The C-MOS switch which switches the coil alternately from battery positive to battery negative has a significant internal resistance and reduce the maximum power output.
− If the Class D receiver is operated at its performance limit then additional disturbing frequencies can occur due to the sampling of 100 kHz.

5 Acoustic modifications

The trend in the hearing instrument world is clear. More and more, hearing instruments are electronic, digital, programmable units. With this emphasis on the electronic characteristics of hearing instruments, it is easy to forget that they also have acoustic properties. Like a musical instrument, if the acoustic quality of a hearing instrument is poor, no amount of complicated electronics can make up for this.

In this chapter, it will be demonstrated how a hearing instrument frequency response can often be quite simply changed for better or worse through acoustic modifications to the microphone, the receiver (hook) or to the earmold. These modifications can also be used by the hearing healthcare professional to a certain extent.

5.1 Acoustic modifications to the microphone

For a discussion of the types of microphones used in hearing instruments, the reader is referred to chapter 4.1.3.

Microphone tubing

The choice of the microphone tubing (length/diameter) determines to a large extent the frequency response. (Figures 5.1 and 5.2)

Length

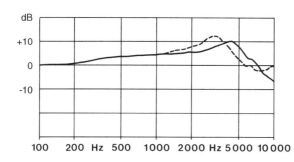

—— Microphone tubing: 2 mm
- - - Microphone tubing: 10 mm
Figure 5.1: Microphone frequency response with different tubing lengths

Lengthening the microphone tube causes a shift in the resonance to lower frequencies

Diameter

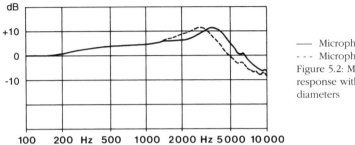

—— Microphone tubing: 1.0 mm
- - - Microphone tubing: 0.5 mm
Figure 5.2: Microphone frequency response with different tubing diameters

Reduction in tubing diameter cuts the high frequencies. The disadvantage of modifying the frequency response in this manner is that it does not diminish noise in the hearing instrument as is the case when the frequency response is altered electronically.

5.2 Acoustic modification by the hearing instrument receiver/hook

The manufacturers of hearing instruments offer a variety of receivers in terms of size, output capability and frequency response. The standard receiver exhibits pronounced resonances; therefore damped receivers are available which suppress the receiver resonances by means of an acoustic filter (damper). In the case of the undamped frequency response of a behind-the-ear receiver, five typical peaks (resonances) can be identified (Figure 5.3).

1. First sound tubing resonance at about 1200 Hz.
2. Receiver resonance at about 2500 Hz.
3. Sound tubing resonance at about 3600 Hz.
4. Sound tubing resonance at about 4800 Hz.
5. Receiver resonance at about 6000 Hz.

dB SPL Output

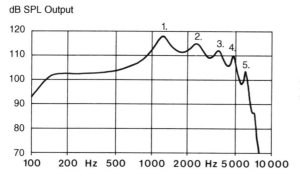

Figure 5.3: Resonance peaks of an undamped receiver

The exact location of the resonance peaks over the whole frequency band depends on the size of the receiver as well as the length and the diameter of the tubing. Hearing instruments with such strong resonances are often experienced by users as sounding unnatural and having an unpleasant tonal quality. Damping of these resonances is often a good way to promote user acceptance of the hearing instrument.

The most frequent and simplest acoustic modification to the behind-the-ear unit is changing the hearing instrument hook. These tubing/receiver resonances can now be damped by means of special filters in the hook (Figure 5.4).

dB SPL Output

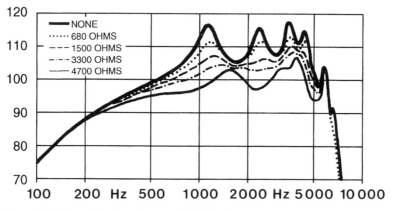

Figure 5.4: Various damping elements in the hook

The advantage of such a flat frequency response obtained by damping of the re-sonances–apart from a natural sound–is the fact that, by smoothing the frequency response, no resonance peaks exceed the discomfort level (UCL). The dynamics of the hearing instrument must not be unnecessarily reduced by this.
It is interesting to note that not only the flow resistance of the damping element but also the placing (in the hook or the earmold) is of great importance.
Figure 5.5 shows various frequency responses measured with the same filter. Varying the position of the filter changes the frequency response.

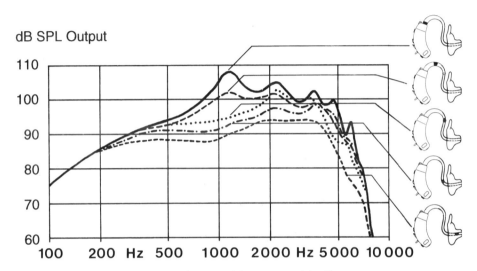

Figure 5.5: Frequency responses as a function of the position of the filter

If the filter is located near to the receiver, the overall response is smoothed slight-ly. When the filter is moved nearer the earmold, a greater overall damping oc-curs. There is an especially large reduction of the output at the first tubing resonance. By careful dimensioning of the hook with the correct filter, a so-called etymotic frequency response is produced.

Etymotic frequency response

By damping the resonance peak at 1000 Hz with a hearing instrument hook, an etymotic frequency response is produced. An etymotic frequency response com-pensates for the loss of the natural auditory canal resonance.

dB SPL Output

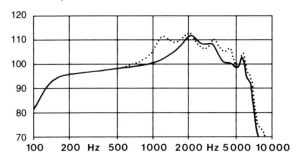

Figure 5.6: Etymotic frequency response with the help of a damping element

Special hooks

The company Etymotic Research manufactures specially shaped hooks which, when combined with commercially-available behind-the-ear instruments, offer simple and effective solutions for fitting three different types of hearing loss. However, these hooks are costly and rather large, limiting their use to only the more serious cases.

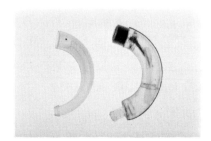

Figure 5.7: Standard hook and special hook (Etymotic Research)

High-tone hook

A high-tone hook makes it possible to alter the response of a broadband hearing instrument such that gain is limited to the high frequency range, dropping sharply for frequencies below 3 kHz (Figure 5.8).

dB Gain

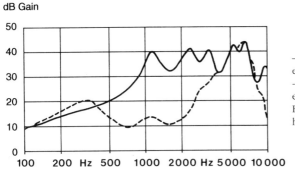

——— Standard hook with normal earmold
- - - High-tone hook with Lybarger earmold
Figure 5.8: Frequency band with high-tone hook

Low-tone hook

This hook has been developed for low frequency hearing losses. The frequency transmission falls sharply after 800 Hz (Figure 5.9).

dB Gain

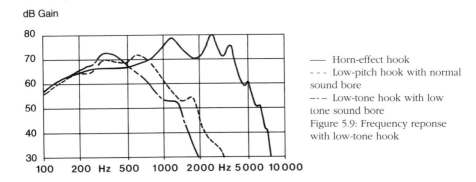

——— Horn-effect hook
- - - Low-pitch hook with normal sound bore
—·— Low-tone hook with low tone sound bore
Figure 5.9: Frequency reponse with low-tone hook

Notch filter hook

The notch filter hook contains a narrow band stop filter which achieves a damping of 20 dB at 2 kHz.
The advantage of such a notch filter is that it can be used with a normal earmold. Thus the effect can be immediately tested in the fitting situation (Figure 5.10).

dB Gain

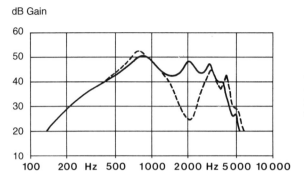

—— Standard hook
- - - Notch filter hook
Figure 5.10: Frequency response
with notch filter hook

5.3 Acoustic modifications to the earmold

The most important acoustic modification which the hearing healthcare professional can carry out is to change the earmold. The question now poses itself as to how and in what frequency range an acoustic modification is possible. Figure 5.11 clearly shows the frequency ranges which can be affected by earmold venting, damping and horn bore.

Important: As the three ranges only slightly overlap, one or more modifications can be made simultaneously.

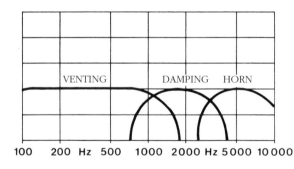

Figure 5.11: Influence of acoustic
modifications on the earmold

Venting

A vent is an additional opening in the earmold leading to the outside air. A vent has various effects according to its size and length.

1) Pressure equalization and elimination of the occlusion effect

Occlusion of the auditory canal causes a considerable increase in loudness for bone-conducted sound, including sounds made by the wearer (own voice, chewing noises). Some sounds (e.g. vocalization) can be amplified as much as 30–40 dB at around 125 Hz due to ear canal occlusion.

In contrast to a sensation of pressure, which can be relieved by drilling a small additional hole in the earmold, the occlusion effect can only be remedied by means of a fully open earmold (Figure 5.12). In fact, reducing the diameter of vents will result in attenuation of signals below 750 Hz yet still allow amplification of up to 20 dB at 1 kHz. In the case of binaural fitting the occlusion effect must be taken into consideration.

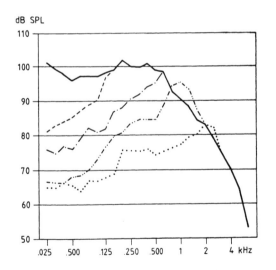

—— Closed earmold
- - - 1 mm vent
—·— 2 mm vent
—··– 3 mm vent
······· open ear canal
Figure 5.12: Influence of vent diameter on the occlusion effect [4]

2) Damping of the low frequencies

By enlarging the size of the vent, gain in the low frequencies is lost. The reduction in gain in the lower frequencies is a function of the diameter and the length of the vent (Figures 5.13/5.14).

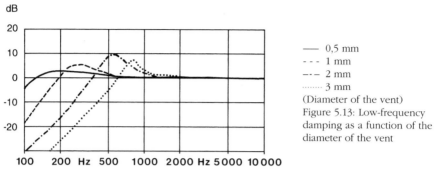

dB

— 0,5 mm
- - - 1 mm
—·— 2 mm
········ 3 mm
(Diameter of the vent)
Figure 5.13: Low-frequency
damping as a function of the
diameter of the vent

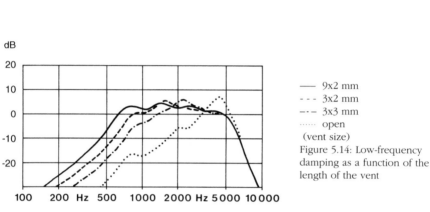

dB

— 9x2 mm
- - - 3x2 mm
—·— 3x3 mm
······ open
(vent size)
Figure 5.14: Low-frequency
damping as a function of the
length of the vent

Avoiding excessive low frequency amplification can improve speech understanding, especially in low frequency noise situations. Changes in the low frequency response of the hearing instrument can be effected either by acoustic or
electrical means. Leaving the ear canal open to some extent is an acoustic modification which can result in up to 30 dB less gain at 500 Hz. Although the same
effect can also be produced with electronic filters, subjective comparisons with
acoustic modifications show a clear preference (both with respect to resultant
sound quality as well as speech understanding) for the acoustic solution.

Damping

By using acoustic damping elements (acoustic resistances) in the earmold, frequencies in the range from 800 Hz to 4000 Hz can be damped (See Page 89). Today these damping elements are usually inserted in the hearing instrument hook rather than the earmold (as it is simpler to do it).

Horn bore

By progressively increasing the earmold bore diameter, the high frequency transmission is positively affected (horn effect). Typical earmolds with a horn bore include, for example, Libby horn and Bakke horn. The effects of various horn bore diameters are shown in Figure 5.15.

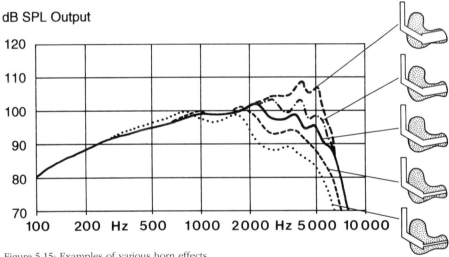

Figure 5.15: Examples of various horn effects

As a rule, the best high frequency transmission as possible is desirable. Problems with horn bores include the relatively large space requirements and the danger of feedback.

5.4 Modifications of feedback

What is feedback?

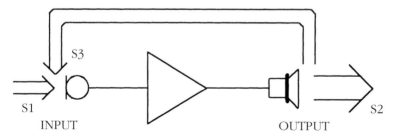

Figure 5.16: Origin of acoustical feedback

1. An input signal S1 is introduced to a system and is amplified.
2. An output signal S2 appears. S2 is larger than S1 by the amplification factor.
3. Part of S2 (signal S3) is fed back to the input (unintentionally). This results in a loop where part of the output signal is continually reintroduced as input to the system and amplified.
→ If S3 is greater than S1 → there is feedback.

What types of feedback are there?

There are 4 different types of feedback in hearing instruments.

1) Acoustic feedback

The most important and frequently occuring kind of feedback is acoustic feedback in which the loop is between the receiver and the microphone. This kind of feedback is often due to a problem with the earmold (vent is too large or there is a poor seal). It is, however, possible that the feedback is due to internal coupling between the microphone and receiver in the hearing instrument, in which case the service engineer must replace the internal microphone and receiver tubes.

2) Mechanical feedback

This appears when the vibrational damping of the microphone and receiver mountings is not adequate. Vibrations which are produced by the receiver are transmitted via the hearing instrument housing and picked up and amplified by the microphone. Mechanical feedback appears with very low frequency hearing instruments and mostly at frequencies below 1000 Hz.

3) Magnetic feedback

Magnetic feedback occurs when the induction coil is active. The magnetic field of the receiver is picked up by the induction coil and again amplified. Magnetic feedback can appear over the hearing instrument's whole frequency range.

4) Electrical feedback

In the case of electrical feedback, the amplifier becomes unstable, most often because of a weak battery. The voltage of the battery decreases and the inner resistance increases, resulting in a low frequency hum, which is referred to as "motor boating" due to its resemblance to the sound of a running motor boat.

Elimination of feedback

In this section, the elimination of acoustic feedback will be discussed. Mechanical, magnetic and electrical feedback can be considered as hearing instrument faults requiring the instrument to be sent to repair by the manufacturer. To eliminate feedback, the following measures must be taken:

a) Determine the type of feedback (Point 1, 2, 3 or 4)

b) In the case of acoustic feedback, one must determine whether it is an external (via the earmold) or an internal (in the hearing instrument housing) type of feedback.
If the hearing instrument hook is closed, the hearing instrument should not whistle. If it does, this means there is internal feedback.

c) Determination of the feedback frequency in the case of acoustic feedback.

1. If the feedback appears at low frequencies (1000 Hz to 2000 Hz) the following measures can eliminate it:
   – reduce the gain
   – damping by means of a filter in the hook of behind-the-ear units
   – reduction of the size of the vent
2. If the feedback appears at high frequencies (3000 Hz to 5000 Hz):
   – reduce the high frequency amplification by means of a high-cut filter or by modifying the earmold
   – reduction of the size of the vent

See also section 8: Hearing instrument troubleshooting

6 Hearing instrument functions

In this chapter the various hearing instrument functions will be detailed more thoroughly. The various functions are for the use of either the hearing health-care professional or the wearer.

6.1 Filter functions

The frequency response can be changed in most hearing instruments. To allow this, an electrical filter is built into the hearing instrument amplifier. These filters are usually manufactured from the electronic components R (resistors), and C (capacitors).

In order to be able to change the frequency response of the hearing instrument, the resistor is replaced by a trimmer (adjustable resistor). The hearing health-care professional needs only a small screwdriver to alter the resistance value and thus match the hearing instrument's frequency response to the hearing loss. The filter can be effective in high or low frequency ranges.

The high pass filter (low cut)

A high pass filter allows, as the name suggests, the higher frequencies to pass unattenuated through the filter.

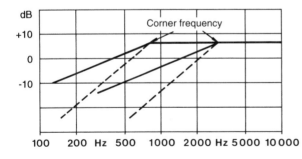

Figure 6.1: High pass filter function

By changing the resistance value, the corner frequencies are changed. The order of the filter indicates the slope of the filter curve.

First order → slope = 6 dB/octave.
Second order → slope = 12 dB/octave.

First order filters are usually so-called passive filters. That is, the filter function is achieved solely through an RC-component. Higher order filters (second to fourth order) will often be active filters. These filters also have active parts (amplifiers) in addition to the passive components (R and C).

The advantage of active filters as compared to passive ones is that active filters can cover a greater frequency range. Modern hearing instruments (particulary digitally progammable units) all have active filters.

Low pass filter (high cut)

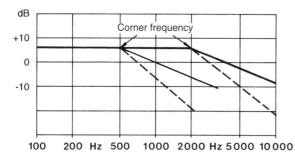

Figure 6.2: Low pass filter function

A low pass filter allows low frequencies to pass unattenuated through the filter. Since most hearing instruments are lacking in high frequency gain (too narrow a receiver band), the low pass filter is mostly used when there is a feedback problem. However, a lowpass filter can also be of help during a new wearer's acclimitization to the hearing instrument. Since the hearing-impaired have not heard the high frequencies for years (or decades), most hearing instruments are initially experienced as sounding too shrill.

The low pass filter can be used to reduce gain in the higher frequencies which can make the hearing instrument easier for the new wearer to accept. The frequency response of the hearing instrument can be widened as the wearer becomes accustomed to again being able to hear high frequency sounds. Research has not demonstrated any immediate improvement in speech understanding subsequent to fitting with a hearing instrument with a wideband frequency response. However, speech understanding scores have been shown to improve significantly after a couple of months of hearing instrument use.

6.2 Output limiting

Output limiting plays an important role during the fitting. It prevents the maximum output sound pressure from exceeding the discomfort level of the wearer. There are a number of different ways of limiting the maximum output sound pressure. The decision as to which method of output limiting is most appropriate in a given case must be made by the hearing healthcare professional together with the hearing-impaired individual.

There is no single type of limiter that is optimal for every kind of hearing loss.

6.2.1 The peak clipper

In the block diagram (Figure 6.3) is a simple presentation of output limitation by means of peak clipping (PC).

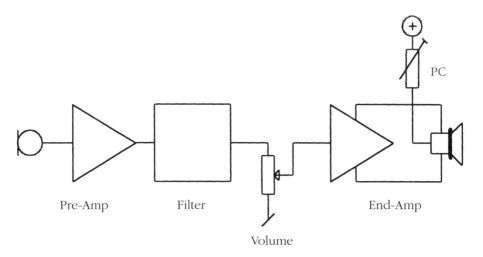

Figure 6.3: Block diagram of a PC limiter (Class B)

A peak clipper, as its name suggests, "clips" the peaks of the signal that exceed a certain voltage.

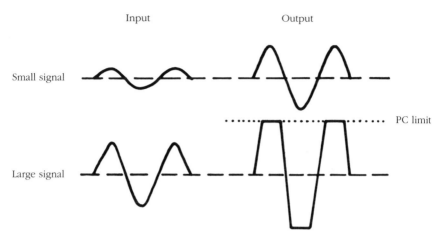

Figure 6.4: Operation of a PC with various input signals

Limiting of the output sound pressure by peak clipping leads to a large amount of distortion. Since the peak clipper works very quickly, there is virtually no delay in the effect. PC is suitable for the hearing-impaired wearer with a limited dynamic range (requiring a great deal of gain, but having a relatively low uncomfortable loudness level). The method of operation of a PC is shown in the input/output function (Figure 6.5).

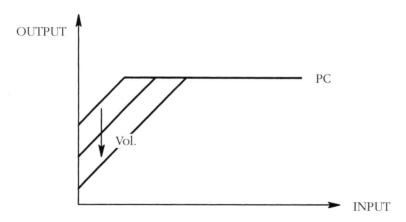

Figure 6.5: Input/output function with PC limiting

The maximum sound pressure never exceeds the limit set by the PC. The PC limit is not changed by reducing gain via the volume control. As the gain is reduced, a greater sound pressure level is required before the hearing instrument goes into saturation and peak clipping occurs. The kneepoint on the input/output graph moves to the right (greater input level).

Advantages and disadvantages of a PC

+ Peak clipping is the means of output limitation allowing the greatest possible amplification. (There is no gain reduction when limiting is reached.)
+ Acts instantaneously (No attack and release time)
− Results in a great deal of distortion

A special kind of PC is diode compression.

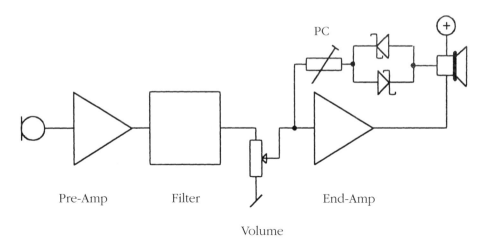

Figure 6.6: Circuit diagram of a diode compression

Antiparallel diodes are connected across the final stage. These limit the signal to a maximum of one diode voltage (300 mV by using Schottky diodes). The diode compression is especially used with Class A output amplifiers. Previously, a resistor in series with the receiver was used (asymetrical peak clipping), but this resulted in a great deal of second harmonic distortion which is detrimental to speech understanding. The diode compression (symmetrical peak clipping) reduced the amount of second harmonic distortion.

6.2.2 The AGC circuit

AGC = Automatic Gain Control

AGC circuits alter the amplification as soon as a certain level (kneepoint, AGC threshold) is reached. As long as these levels are not attained, the AGC functions as a linear amplifier.

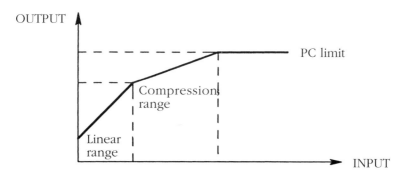

Figure 6.7: Input/output function of an AGC circuit

If the kneepoint is reached, the AGC begins to reduce its amplification. → It enters the compression range.

The compression ratio can be predetermined by the hearing instrument designer. A compression ratio of 2:1 means that the input signal must be increased by 2 parts in order to increase the output signal by one part (dB-scale).

If the AGC has a very high compression ratio (10:1 or more) then it can be utilized as a limiter.

The compression ratio is dependent on time constants. The steady state condition (measured according to standard) indicates the compression ratio. Dynamic AGC activation (e.g. during speech) reduces the compression ratio when attack and release times are too long.

Unlike the peak clipper, the AGC circuit needs time to react

The time it takes the AGC to decrease the gain to the limiting level is called the attack time. Once the AGC is in operation and the input SPL is no longer high enough to require limiting, the time it takes for the hearing instrument to resume normal gain function is called the release time (see chapter [3.2.8]). Attack and release times are not set arbitrarily but are dependent on which functions the AGC possesses; that is, what type of hearing-impairment is to be fitted.

AGC circuits are divided into two types which are designed for different applications.

AGCi and AGCo

a) The AGCi circuit

AGCi = Automatic Gain Control Input

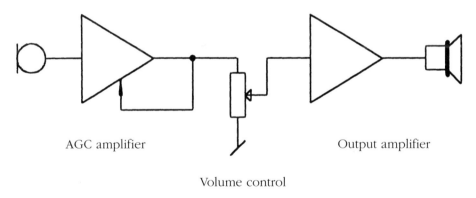

AGC amplifier

Volume control

Output amplifier

Figure 6.8: Diagram of an AGCi circuit

An AGCi is defined as one where the AGC circuit is located before the volume control (potentiometer), so that the AGC circuit is activated by the input SPL. The operation of an AGCi circuit is clearly illustrated by the input/output function.

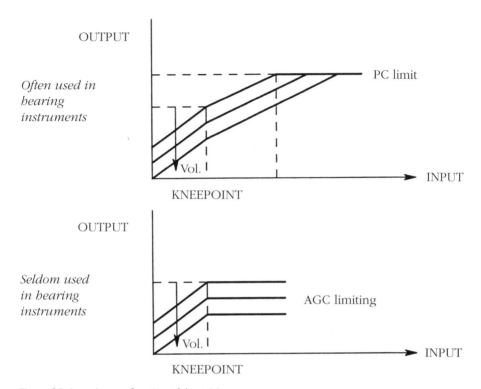

OUTPUT

*Often used in
hearing
instruments*

PC limit

Vol.

KNEEPOINT

INPUT

OUTPUT

*Seldom used
in hearing
instruments*

AGC limiting

Vol.

KNEEPOINT

INPUT

Figure 6.9: Input/output function of the AGCi

In an AGCi circuit, the input SPL required to activate the circuit remains constant even with a reduction in gain via the volume control. Since the AGCi usually has a compression ratio of only 2:1 or 3:1, the maximum output sound pressure must be limited by either a PC or an AGCo with a high compression ratio.

The AGCi (e.g compression ratio 2:1) is often used in cases where recruitment is a major problem for the wearer. In order to preserve good speech under-standing, fast attack and release times are crucial. This means that syllabic compression must be provided which again indicates fast attack and release times. When AGCi is used as a syllabic compressor, attack time should be less than 10 ms and release time less than 50 ms.

The disadvantages of the AGCi utilized in this manner are harmonic distortions at low frequencies and, because of the controlling effects, a noisy hearing in-strument (pumping).

The AGCi is seldom used today for output limiting since gain reduction via the volume control also reduces the output SPL by the same value.

b) The AGCo

AGCo = Automatic Gain Control output

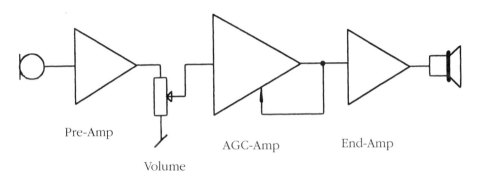

Figure 6.10: Schematic drawing of an AGCo circuit

An AGCo is defined as one where the AGC circuit is positioned after the volume control.

A characteristic of an AGCo circuit is that the kneepoint of the AGCo moves to the right (greater input SPL) on reduction of amplification via the volume control. The result is a large range of linear amplification.

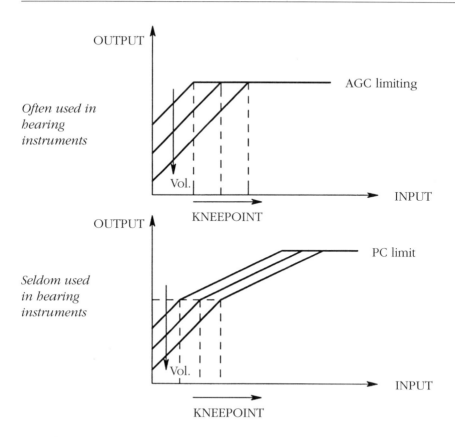

Figure 6.11: Input/output function of the AGCo

Today the AGCo is largely used for output limiting (compression ratio > 10:1) which has the advantage of little distortion even at maximum sound pressure in the hearing instrument. In other words, in a hearing instrument with an AGCo as output limiter, there is never more than 10% distortion under any operating conditions. When used for this kind of output limiting, the AGCo should have an attack time of < 10 ms. The release time is about 200 ms. This also leads to the so-called "pumping effect". In order to prevent this, an adaptive release time is used which can range from 50 ms to 1,5 s depending on how long the AGC circuit is activated. An AGCo with a compression ratio as low as 2:1 or 3:1 is scarcely used anymore.

7 Hearing instrument accessories and features

This chapter details a number of options in conjunction with hearing instruments.

7.1 Induction coil

An induction coil is built into nearly all behind-the-ear units and some in-the-ear units. The induction coil is operational when the input selection switch is on the "T" setting.
This coil picks up electromagnetic signals and converts them into an electrical voltage which is then amplified by the hearing instrument.

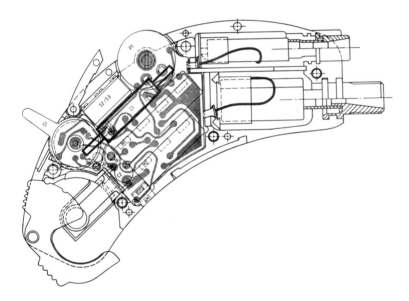

Figure 7.1: Hearing instrument with induction coil

The name "telecoil" derives from the fact that it picks up electromagnetic signals from the telephone, making it possible to use the T setting for telephoning. Unfortunately, the magnetic field radiated from a modern telephone is much weaker than with old telephones so that the signal is often too weak.
The main purpose of the induction coil in hearing instruments is the reception of magnetic fields from special induction loops. Such loop systems are common in churches and public buildings. The advantage of these loop systems is that the hearing instrument receives and amplifies the signal (e.g. the pastor) and not the surrounding noise (See also chapter [3.2.7] 'Induction coil measurement').

7.2 The audio input

Many behind-the-ear units are equipped with an audio input. The usual abbreviation for audio input is "A".

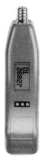
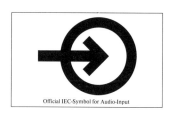

Official IEC-Symbol for Audio-Input

Figure 7.2: Behind the ear unit with audio input and audio input symbol

Before it became useful for CROS and BiCROS applications, the audio input had a quite definite aim:

To pick up an acoustic or audio signal directly and undistorted from the signal source. When listening to speech, there is no loss of the high frequency speech components and background noise is not picked up. All audio units (e.g. television, radio) could be connected electrically via a cable connection or acoustically via a microphone directly to the loudspeaker.

The audio input consists of electrical contacts to which a plug or an audio shoe can be connected.

Electrically, the audio input:
a) is in parallel with the microphone
b) is in parallel with the induction coil
c) has a separate preamplifier

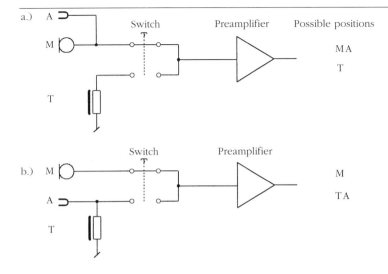

Figure 7.3: Different electrical circuits for the audio input

7.2.1 CROS

CROS: Contralateral Routing Of Signals

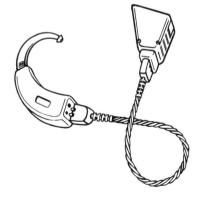

Figure 7.4: CROS adaptor

Design

a) The CROS design seen most frequently today is that used in conjunction with spectacle frames. The microphone is removed from the hearing instrument and attached to the bow opposite the hearing instrument. The microphone is connected via a thin 3-core cable to the existing microphone terminals of the amplifier.

b) (Without spectacles)
The hearing instrument microphone is removed from the hearing instrument. A CROS adaptor, resembling a small BTE unit and normally containing only a microphone, is placed behind the contralateral ear and connected to the audio input via a thin cable.

Purpose

– A CROS solution can often allow an open ear fitting.
– In the case of particularly severe hearing loss, increased amplification is possible (without feedback).
– Only one ear receives amplification but information to be heard often comes from the other side (e.g. taxi driver).

7.2.2 BICROS

Design

The same as for CROS, but with a microphone in the hearing instrument as well. This means that there is a microphone on both sides of the head but only one ear being fitted.

Purpose

The worst ear cannot be fitted. → The patient hears from both sides.
Important: BICROS is not a binaural fitting.

7.2.3 The hand-held microphone

The hand-held microphone is designed to allow the hearing-impaired listener to be closer to the speaker (→ better signal/noise ratio). The hand-held microphone is connected via a cable to the audio input enabling better understanding under noisy conditions, especially if the hand-held microphone has good directional characteristics.

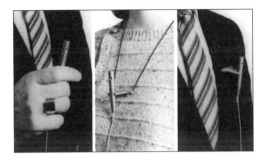

Figure 7.5: Hand-held microphone

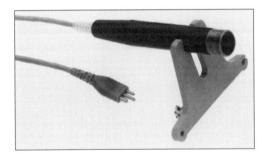

Frequently, the hand-held microphone is used when fitting children. For example, a hand-held microphone makes it possible for a mother to communicate with her hearing-impaired child as well as to train speech and language skills without the interference of ambient noises. A hearing instrument microphone is frequently built into the hand-held housing in order to obtain a similar frequency response to that of the microphone in the wearer's hearing instrument.

7.2.4 FM system

An FM system (FM = Frequency Modulation) consists of a microphone (frequently a directional microphone), an FM transmitter and an FM receiver. It is suitable both for group amplification systems in schools (i.e. an FM transmitter and several FM receivers) as well as for personal use in meetings and conferences (the speaker has an FM transmitter; the hearing-impaired listeners have FM receivers that are tuned to the same predetermined frequency). Because the microphone picks up the speech directly from the speaker, the speaking distance is less than 20 cm. Wireless FM systems possess good speech transmission properties.

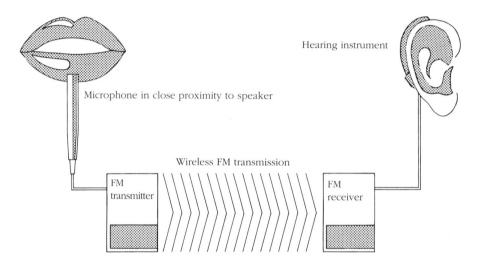

Figure 7.6: Operating principle of an FM system

The FM receiver is connected to the audio input of the hearing instrument. The purpose of an FM system is the same as for the hand-held microphone: to bring the speaker closer to the ear; that is, to improve signal/noise ratio. FM systems work with various transmission frequencies. The following transmitting frequencies are assigned according to country:
– France: 36–39 MHz and 175–176 MHz
– Germany: 36–39 MHz and 173–175 MHz
– Switzerland: 36–39 MHz and 174–223 MHz
– USA: 72–76 MHz and 216–217 MHz.

If several FM systems are being used simultaneously in a building, different transmission frequencies must be used in the different rooms to avoid mutual interference.
Important: It is possible to serve many receivers with one transmitter [teacher (transmitter) and pupil (receiver)]. It is not possible to work with several transmitters and one receiver (different teachers and one student). → The receiver will only receive one transmitter, namely the strongest.

7.3 Remote control

Remote control has long been popular in home electronics. There is hardly a television on the market today which does not have a remote control. Remote controls with hearing instruments are only possible through the incorporation of complex integrated circuits. Various hearing instrument manufacturers offer different types of remote controls.

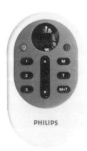

Infrared

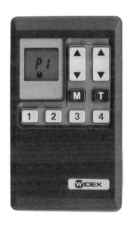

Radio (FM)

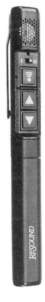

Ultrasonic

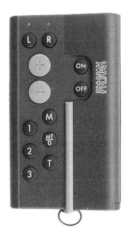

Inductive

Figure 7.7: Different remote control systems

All remote controls can alter the gain of the hearing instrument. More complex remote controls (and hearing instruments) have additional functions such as:
– Switching from M/MT/T
– Different user programs
– ON/OFF function
– Display

An important difference between the various remote controls is the method of transmission employed. Today, there are 4 means of transmission in hearing instrument remote controls:
a) Ultrasonic
b) Infrared
c) Radio (FM)
d) Inductive

Advantages and disadvantages of the various transmission systems

a) Ultrasonic
+ Receiver (microphone) is already in the hearing instrument.
– Remote control is only possible with line of sight. Otherwise there is too much interference. → No binaural control is possible.

b) Infrared
+ Less sensitive to interference. Proven remote control technology.
– Remote control is only possible with line of sight. → No binaural control is possible.

c) Radio (FM)
+ Good transmission properties, no line of sight necessary → binaural control possible
– Sensitive to interference from strong magnetic fields (PC)

d) Inductive
+ Good transmission properties, no line of sight necessary → binaural control possible
– Sensitive to interference from strong magnetic fields (PC)

7.4 Batteries

The battery is the power supply of the hearing instrument. It is a 'galvanic voltage source'. What is a galvanic voltage source?

If two dissimilar metal plates (e.g. a copper and a zinc plate) are immersed in an
electrically conducting fluid (electrolyte), a voltage develops across the two
plates.

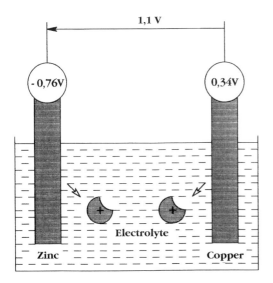

Figure 7.8: Galvanic voltage source

Positive metal ions pass into the fluid from the surface of a metal immersed in
the electrolyte so that the remaining metal becomes negatively charged with respect to the fluid. The charge varies depending on the mass of the ions released.
Precious metals are dissolved less than nonprecious metals. When two dissimilar metal plates are immersed in the same electrolyte, they become charged dif-
ferently so that there is a potential difference between the two plates. If the plates
are connected, the potential difference causes a current to flow between them.
Because the precious metal is less strongly negatively charged than the nonprecious metal, the precious metal constitutes the positive (plus) pole and the nonprecious metal the negative (minus) pole of the voltage source. In this way, a
galvanic element results. The metals are arranged in such a way that each one
is positive with respect to the preceding one so as to give an electrochemical
series of the metals.

An example of an electrochemical series

Aluminium	– 1.70 V	Tin	– 0.14 V	Carbon	+ 0.74 V
Zinc	– 0.76 V	Lead	– 0.12 V	Silver	+ 0.80 V
Chrome	– 0.56 V	Hydrogen	0.00 V	Mercury	+ 0.85 V
Iron	– 0.54 V	Copper	+ 0.35 V	Gold	+ 1.50 V

Example

The zinc-carbon element is widely used in pocket flashlights and other portable electrical appliances. If we consider the electrochemical series, we find:
Zinc   – 0.76 V
Carbon + 0.74 V
thus there results an initial voltage of 1.5 V between the two metals.

In the case of hearing instrument batteries, packing density (the highest capacity in the smallest space) is of extreme importance. Therefore, other materials are used. Today, so-called dry batteries are used; these differ from those described above in that the electrolyte has been thickened into a paste.

Size

There are 5 standard sizes available:

a) '675'
Largest of the batteries used in hearing instruments today. Used in large and powerful behind-the-ear units.

b) '13'
Same thickness as the '675' but smaller in diameter. Used in smaller behind-the-ear units and powerful concha units.

c) '312'
Same diameter as the '13' but thinner. Used in in-the-ear units.

d) 'A10'
Same thickness as the '312' but smaller in diameter. Used in small canal units.

e) 'A5'
Same diameter as the 'A10' but thinner. Used in the CIC (completely in the canal) units.

Chemistry

Button batteries work on the basis of mercuric oxide or on the basis of zinc-air. Silver oxide batteries have a higher voltage (1.5 V), but are hardly used anymore because of their high price.

Circuit technology

The battery represents a voltage source. However, it is not ideal in that it has an internal resistance which is in series with the voltage source. The older the battery is, the greater is this internal resistance. If the internal resistance becomes too great it can have negative effects on the hearing instrument (more distortion, humming etc.). The magnitude of the problem depends on the circuit requirements in the hearing instrument.

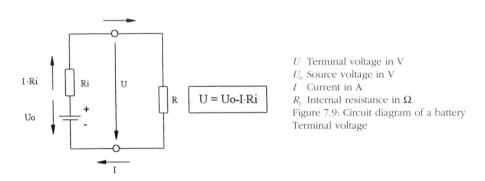

U Terminal voltage in V
U_o Source voltage in V
I Current in A
R_i Internal resistance in Ω
Figure 7.9: Circuit diagram of a battery
Terminal voltage

$$U = U_o - I \cdot R_i$$

7.4.1 Mercury battery

The mercury battery has been the most frequently used battery in hearing instruments, but is now being replaced by the environmentally friendly zinc-air batteries in many countries.

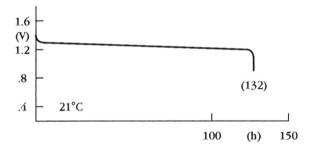

625 Ohms 16 hours per day
Performance in hours
Figure 7.10: Discharge curve of
a 675 mercury battery

The capacity of a '675' mercury battery is about 270 mAh.
The capacity of a '13' mercury battery is about 100 mAh.
The capacity of a '312' mercury battery is about 60 mAh.
The capacity of a 'A10' mercury battery is about 30 mAh.

Advantages and disadvantages of mercury batteries

+ Good quality, long shelf life
+ Stable voltage, small inner resistance, can supply large current
+ Best button batteries
− Environmentally damaging because of large mercury content
− Lower capacity than zinc-air battery

7.4.2 Zinc-air battery

The zinc-air battery has a large capacity and no mercury. The battery has several air holes which are closed by plastic adhesive. When the battery is to be used, the adhesive is removed. Air then enters the battery and the chemical process begins; that is, the battery voltage rises to the unloaded initial value of 1.4 V.
By opening the air holes, the zinc-air battery has a permanent discharge current of about 50 μA, depending on the size of the air holes. The larger the holes, the higher the discharge current. Once a zinc-air battery has been opened, the chemical process cannot be stopped by closing the air holes again. The maximum current that the battery can deliver is also dependent on the size of the air holes.

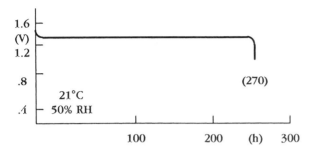

625 Ohms 16 hours per day
Performance in hours
Figure 7.11: Discharge curve of
zinc-air battery

The capacity of a '675' zinc-air battery is about 540 mAh.
The capacity of a '13' zinc-air battery is about 230 mAh.
The capacity of a '312' zinc-air battery is about 110 mAh.
The capacity of a 'A10' zinc-air battery is about 55 mAh.
The capacity of a 'A5' zinc-air battery is about 35 mAh.

Advantages and disadvantages of zinc-air batteries

+ Environmentally friendly
+ Large capacity
− Often not very good quality
− Not very long shelf life
− Continuous discharge current
− Peak current smaller than that of mercury batteries → not suitable for high-performance units

Note: At the end of 1993, prototypes for new zinc-air batteries had been developed which should be able to provide enough power for high performance units as well! These new batteries may well prove amazing.

8 Hearing instrument troubleshooting

When a hearing instrument is returned as defective, there are a number of tests that can be performed without having to open the unit.

8.1 Feedback
8.1.1 Feedback from an ITE

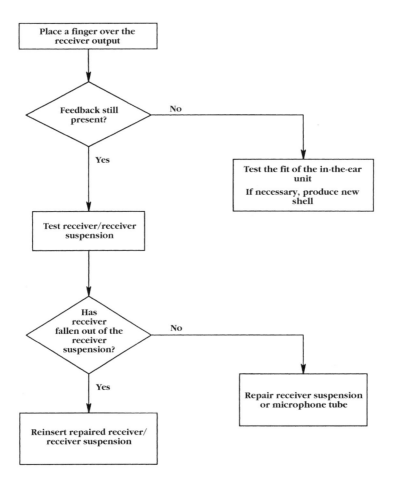

Figure 8.1: Troubleshooting of an ITE with acoustical feedback

8.1.2 Feedback from a BTE

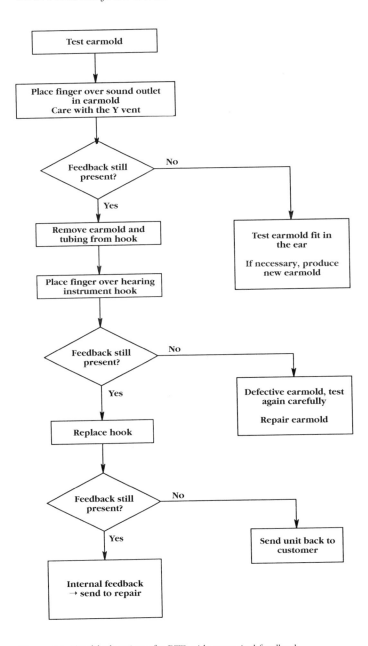

Figure 8.2: Troubleshooting of a BTE with acoustical feedback

8.2 The unit does not amplify the acoustic signal!

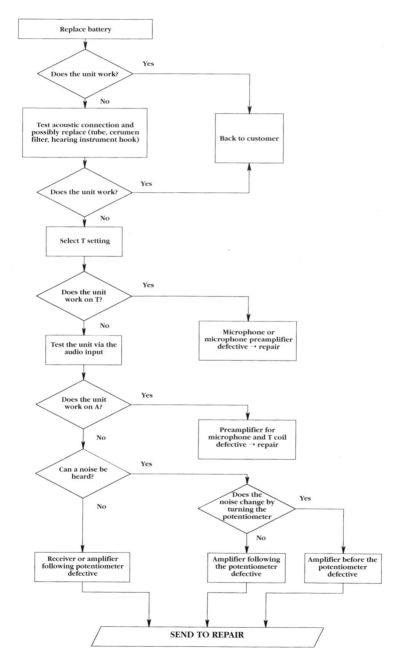

Figure 8.3: Troubleshooting of a hearing instrument

9 Digitally programmable hearing instruments

Hearing instrument technology has changed greatly over the past few years. At first, the focus was on the improvement and miniaturization of the electronic components. Great strides were made in developing better sound transducers. It has been possible to produce microphones with extremely low internal noise as well as receivers with frequency responses of up to 10 kHz.

An additional leap in hearing instrument technology was the introduction of the digitally programmable hearing instrument. No previous development has offered more possibilities for better fitting than the digitally programmable hearing instrument. This chapter presents a discussion of this new generation of instruments.

9.1 What are digitally programmable hearing instruments?

A digitally programmable hearing instrument makes use of a cable connection to a personal computer or a special programming device to manipulate the settings. Via this link, the hearing healthcare professional changes the various parameters of the hearing instrument from the programming unit. Prior to the introduction of digitally programmable hearing instruments, such a high degree of flexibility was unknown. The following are just a few of the parameters which can be changed by a mere press of a button: overall amplification, low frequency amplification, high frequency amplification, maximum output sound pressure, output limiting system (PC or AGC), AGC kneepoint and compression ratio.

Important: Several parameters can be changed and compared simultaneously. The possibility for switching rapidly between various settings allows the hearing instrument wearer to judge which setting best facilitates understanding of speech in noise or which sounds best in quiet surroundings.

Subsequent to fitting of the hearing instrument, the various parameters (amplification, filter coefficients, etc.) can be stored digitally either in the hearing instrument or in the remote control unit, depending on the system. This stored memory will not be lost, even when the hearing instrument's battery is changed.

In the case of a digitally programmable hearing instrument, it is only the settings which are changed and stored digitally. The analog signal is processed using analog principles.

Important: A digitally programmable hearing instrument is not a digital hearing instrument.

The digital hearing instrument utilizes digital signal processing. This means that the analog signal is converted to a digital one and processed digitally.

The hearing healthcare professional can, as a routine follow-up procedure, connect the hearing instrument to the programming device or the computer, read out the stored data and make any necessary alterations in the settings. A further advantage of some programmable hearing instruments is that various settings can be stored as programs in the hearing instrument. This enables the wearer to select the most advantageous setting (usually via a remote control) for any given listening environment. For example, the hearing instrument may have a program for quiet surroundings, another for listening to music (with bass and treble boosting) as well as a program designed to optimize speech understanding under noisy listening conditions.

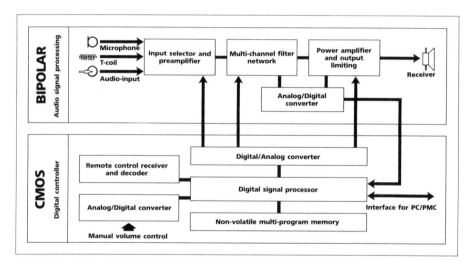

Fig. 9.1: Construction of a digitally programmable hearing instrument

9.2 Programming possibilities

Within the next few years, digitally programmable hearing instruments will gain increasing acceptance on the market. This creates a dilemma for the hearing healthcare professional, who must decide on whether to use a special programming device or a personal computer for fitting these instruments.

9.2.1 Programming devices

At first glance, the simply operated programming devices would appear to be the best–and certainly most straightforward–solution. Hearing healthcare professionals who have no experience with personal computers generally prefer the programming devices initially because they are easily mastered. One of the disadvantages of programming devices is that each hearing instrument manufacturer has its own dedicated programming device, making it necessary for the hearing healthcare professional to have three or four different ones on hand to be able to fit just a few of the instruments on the market.To avoid this, the PMC was developed by Siemens in Erlangen in collaboration with various other hearing instrument manufacturers (Hansaton, Philips, Phonak, Rexton).

PMC

The PMC is a programming device with which hearing instruments from Argosy, Danavox, Hansaton, Philips, Phonak, Rexton, Siemens, Qualiton and 3M can be adjusted. In order to program a hearing instrument, a programming module from the manufacturer of the hearing instrument in question is needed. The module is plugged into the back of the PMC. A maximum of five different modules can be plugged in simultaneously. If an upgrade of the software by the hearing instrument manufacturer is necessary (e.g. for a new hearing instrument), the old module can be easily replaced by the new one, and the system is immediately ready for use again. The PMC has an LCD display of sixteen lines enabling graphical representation of current hearing instrument curves. It is possible to display ear simulator, 2 cc coupler or KEMAR responses. The PMC has two RS 232 C interfaces which make a connection possible to a personal computer or–more frequently–to a printer.

The PMC has the same disadvantages as all other programming devices. These include a poor resolution monochromatic LCD display, too little space for storing clients' data and, especially, limited computer capacity, which precludes complicated adjustment support. Thus the hearing instruments of the future (digital hearing instruments) cannot be adjusted using the PMC.

The PMC can only be a transitional solution. It will ultimately be necessary to utilize a personal computer for hearing instrument fitting.

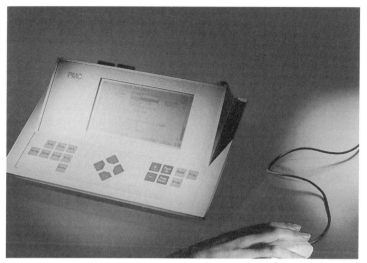

Fig. 9.2: The PMC

9.2.2 The Personal Computer

The personal computer (PC) presents the most complete solution for hearing instrument adjustment. The following components are required for this:
– IBM compatible PC (an at least 386 processor)
– Specific hearing instrument manufacturer interface
– Specific hearing instrument manufacturer adjustment software

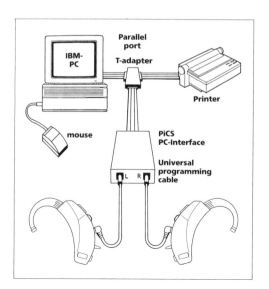

Fig. 9.3: Digitally programmable hearing instruments with personal computer

The PC has none of the disadvantages of the programming devices. The PC offers:
– virtually limitless display possibilities
– adequate storage capacity
– great computer capacity

The PC fulfills all the prerequisites which will be necessary to adjust the digital hearing instruments of the future.

The various programmable hearing instruments can differ enormously from one another, as does their corresponding PC software. In addition, it is necessary to utilize an interface specific to the manufacturer when programming a given hearing instrument. Obviously, it would involve considerable inconvenience and expense for the hearing healthcare professional to be able to fit programmable hearing instruments from different manufacturers. This has been the impetus behind standardization of hardware (interface) and software in the area of programmable hearing instrument fitting.

HIMSA/NOAH/HI-PRO

HIMSA

HIMSA (Hearing Instrument Manufacturer Software Association) is a development association founded by the hearing instrument companies Danavox, Oticon, Phonak and Widex in Denmark in 1993. The objective of HIMSA was to develop a software standard for hearing instrument adjustment (especially for programmable hearing instruments). This software was launched at the end of 1993 under the name NOAH.

NOAH

NOAH is the software platform (in Windows) for the adjustment of programmable hearing instruments. It makes it possible for the hearing healthcare professional to control and manage his whole field of work on the PC with an easily operated program interface. NOAH enables optimal hearing instrument adjustment and programming, as well as efficient management of client data, audiometric data, and administrative affairs.

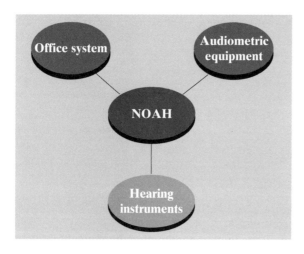

Fig. 9.4: The hearing healthcare professional's work areas with NOAH

The industry standard NOAH allows every manufacturer of hearing instruments, audiometers, office systems, etc. to develop his own modules (software packages) which NOAH then links together. These various modules can then be started from the NOAH platform. What are known as adjustment modules are at the hearing healthcare professional's disposal for the adjustment. These are made available by the hearing instrument manufacturers as separate software and are specially geared to their products' possibilities. Through the direct link between NOAH and an audiometer, the adjusted data can be checked directly "in situ". The following manufacturers have already converted to NOAH standard (as of 1 February, 1995):

Hearing instruments

A&M, Ascom, Audio Service, Bernafon, GN Danavox, Oticon, Phonak, ReSound, Rexton, Rion, Siemens Audiologische Technik, Starkey, Unitron Industries, Viennatone, Widex, 3M.

Audiological metering devices

Acousticon Hörsysteme, Interacoustics, Madsen Electronics, Rexton Danplex.

Office systems

Andis Informatik, Andit Data, Audio Care, IPRO, Pro-Hear.

NOAH requires the following hardware and software:
– IBM compatible PC (minimum 386 processor, 4 MB RAM, 120 MB hard disk, VGA colour monitor
– Windows 3.1 (software)
– Printer equipped for graphics
– Interface (between PC and hearing instrument)

HI-PRO

With NOAH, a standard was developed which allows the hearing healthcare professional to adjust all the various manufacturers' programmable hearing instruments. However, an interface box is still needed to link the PC and hearing instrument. The interface edits the data in such a manner that the PC and hearing instrument can communicate with one another. As mentioned previously, a special interface would be necessary for each hearing instrument manufacturer. Consequently, HI-PRO was developed as a means of saving the hearing healthcare professional the inconvenience and cost of so many devices. HI-PRO is an interface designed by Madsen Electronics for standardization around NOAH, including the requirements of all hearing instrument manufacturers.

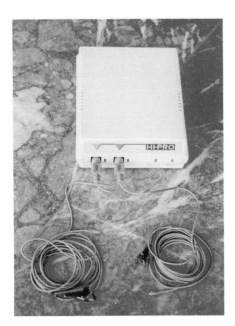

Fig. 9.5: Programming interface HI-PRO

9.3 Advantages and disadvantages of programmable hearing instruments

Although programmable hearing instruments open up a world of possibilities, the new technologies involved made them seem at first to be rather a mixed blessing. Drastic changes were required of both hearing instrument manufacturers as well as fitters to be able to successfully use the new technologies. The manufacturers had to struggle with the usual bugs inherent in new products while the hearing healthcare professionals had to abandon tried and true fitting strategies. Although it has only been a few years since its commercial debut, the advantages of the programmable hearing instrument are already clearly apparent.

1) Advantages for the hearing-impaired user

The benfits of digitally programmable hearing instruments for the wearer are perhaps the most important.

a) Instrument complexity
+ Digitally programmable hearing instruments have much more complex electronics. This means that overload of the instruments is better controlled, resulting in less distortion.
+ There is greater filtering potential, enabling a better fitting for the individual hearing loss.
+ Various sound pressure limiting systems are possible in one unit so that the user can select the one best suited for him.

b) Remote control
+ Binaural control is possible.
+ With remote control, simpler operation of the hearing instrument is possible.
+ It is only with remote control that some functions are possible (e.g. various hearing programs).
+ Users with decreased manual dexterity can easily operate the hearing instrument.

c) User's programs
+ A digitally programmable hearing instrument can have several programs, each of which can be set to amplify and filter the signal in different ways. The user can then select the program best suited for a particular situation (e.g. noise, music, party, etc.).

d) Service

+ Mechanical parts (e.g. trimmers) are replaced by electronic components in the digitally programmable hearing instrument. As a consequence, there is not so much wear and tear on the instrument, making it less prone to need repair.

2) Advantages for the hearing healthcare professional

a) Fitting

+ Simpler programming (no tiny trimmers to be manipulated).
+ "Compare Mode"; instrument settings differing by more than just one trimmer setting can be compared.
+ Two instruments can be adjusted simultaneously.

b) Computer

+ A given setting including the effects of various acoustic parameters (venting, horn, damper, etc.) can be calculated.
+ Storage of fitting data in the client database

10 The digital hearing instrument

10.1 Introduction

In the next few years, an improved understanding of the various kinds of hearing impairments will lead to development of hearing instruments which respond even more specifically to the problems of the hearing-impaired. The problems associated with hearing loss are far more encompassing than just elevated sound detection thresholds. Therefore, hearing instruments must be even more sophisticated if they are to help the user take full advantage of residual hearing. The increase in signal processing complexity necessary for this can be achieved by a digital hearing instrument system which includes both hardware and software. In order to be fully able to exploit the possibilities of digital signal processing in the hearing instrument, new diagnostic and fitting methods are necessary.

10.2 What is digital signal processing?

The decisive characteristic of digital signal processing is the conversion of the continuous time analog signals into sampled discrete time data points (numbers). In Fig. 10.1, the conversion of an analog signal into a digital one is shown.

– The upper curve (a) represents the continuous-time analog signal. The time is shown on the x-axis and the amplitude on the y-axis.
– Curve (b) shows the analog signal once again which is sampled at certain time intervals.
– Curve (c) shows the typical discrete-time digital signal. The sampled numerical values shown are those which are used to create the typical stepped curve.
– (d) shows the (digital) numerical values of the sampled analog signal.

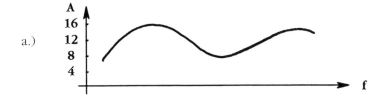

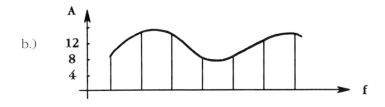

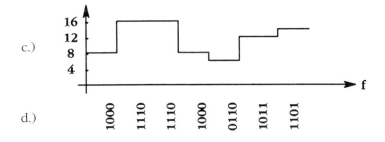

Fig. 10.1: Conversion of an analog signal into a digital one.

The numerical values from (d) are further processed; in digital signal processing, this means that calculations are made with these numerical values.

Fig. 10.2 shows the example of a conversion of an analog signal into a digital one with additional signal processing. The numerical values are multiplied by factor 2 and again converted into an analog signal.

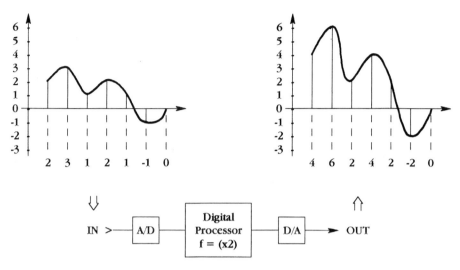

Fig. 10.2: Conversion with signal processing

The result of this multiplication in digital signal processing gives an amplification of the analog signal. In this way, complicated (nonlinear) signal changes are made possible by special computer algorithms. A further advantage is that the algorithms can be changed during signal processing. This means that the arithmetic functions adjust to the input or output signal (adaptive signal processing). Adaptive signal processing is used, for example, in feedback suppression in order to be able to react optimally under changing conditions (e.g. hand on the hearing instrument, chewing).

10.3 Why digital hearing instruments?

Complexity

Increasing the complexity in the design of hearing instruments means greater flexibility and performance capabilities. Because digital technology enables more complex signal processing than analog technology, its advantages grow ever more apparent. While some improvements for simpler hearing instruments can be accomplished using analog technology (e.g. less power consumption), more complex instruments must be of digital construction. In fact, some solutions are simply not possible using analog technology (or only at enormous expense).

Technology

The possibilities of analog technology are practically exhausted. Future potential lies in digital technology. As an example: In the next ten years, analog circuits will become about 20% smaller on the basis of possible technological improvements. In contrast, the degree of miniturization possible with digital circuits is 90%!

10.4 Possibilities and prerequisites for the digital hearing instrument

First and foremost the question arises as to what actual improvements are possible in digital hearing instruments. Certain improvements can be directly implemented based on information already at hand, while others will make necessary a more in-depth audiological diagnostic test battery to optimize success.

Direct improvements

The following solutions can be implemented in a digital hearing instrument without more exact knowledge of the hearing loss. It should always be possible to switch off the individual functions.

10.4.1 Adaptive suppression of the acoustic feedback

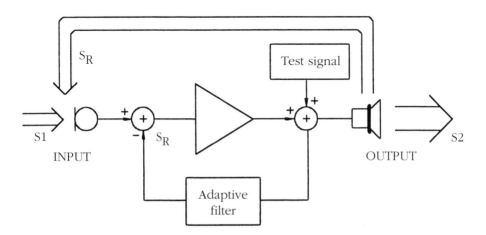

Fig. 10.3: Acoustic feedback suppression

Acoustic feedback represents the greatest limitation in fitting hearing instruments.
– Because of feedback, high frequency amplification is often less than desired, resulting in poorer speech understanding.
– Larger ventilation bores which offer greater wearing comfort can only be used in cases where little gain is needed.

In the case of a suppression of feedback, the feedback path S_R is analysed exactly by means of a test signal. A digital adaptive filter is set in such a manner that an antiphase signal $-S_R$ obliterates the feedback. In this way, the amplification of the instrument can be increased by about 20 dB before any additional acoustic feedback occurs.

At first glance, suppression of the acoustic feedback of more than 50 dB would be desirable, making open mold fittings possible in virtually all cases. However, the suppression has a practical limit. Feedback occurs when the signal S_R, which is fed back from the earphone to the microphone, is just as intense as the input signal $S_1 \rightarrow S_R = S_1$. If feedback is prevented, S_R can be larger than S_1 by the factor of suppression. In the case of too great a suppression of the acoustic feedback, this can have a very disturbing effect on the surroundings (people to whom one is talking) because a loud sound emerges from the ear of the hearing instrument wearer.

10.4.2 Slowing-down of speech

The speech signal is drawn out over time without changing the spectrum (acoustic pattern) in order to facilitate speech understanding. This is possible because the speech is stored. To prevent the slower speech falling too far behind the ongoing signal, pauses in the speech are filled. In the case of a slowing-down of speech, it is not possible to make use of lipreading.

10.4.3 Beam former

It is possible to construct a better directional microphone using at least two microphones and an adaptive digital filter. When directed at the signal source, such microphones have a narrower intake beam than other directional microphones. This would be a particular advantage in understanding speech in noisy surroundings.

Indirect improvements

Additional improvements which are possible with a digital hearing instrument will be described here. Apart from loss of hearing acuity, hearing-impaired persons also suffer from recruitment, reduced summation of loudness and greatly increased frequency masking. As these problems are not indicated on an audiogram, more comprehensive audiological testing is required to optimize fitting of the digital hearing instrument. A digital hearing instrument without adjustment software is inconceivable.

10.4.4 Recruitment

A healthy cochlea is an active system with approx. 50 to 60 dB amplification (control range) measured at threshold. The amplification is regulated nonlinearly by the outer hair cells. The transmission properties of this system can be compared with a compressor. With increasing sound pressure level, the system reduces the amplification continuously (controlled by the outer hair cells)–at high sound pressure levels to nearly 0 dB.

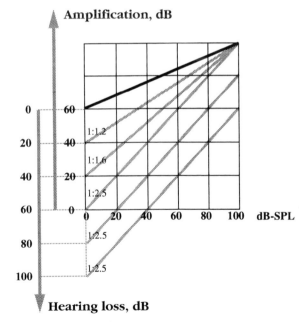

Fig. 10.4: Characteristics of the cochlear amplifier

When the outer hair cells are damaged, cochlear amplification decreases and the regulation process is increasingly lost. Transmission degenerates from a compressive to a linear character. With a hearing loss over 60 dB, the cochlear amplifier is already inactive and the loss of the inner hair cells brings about a further linear shift of the hearing threshold. A maximum compression factor of 2.5:1 suffices as compensation for the loss of the outer hair cells. A digital hearing instrument can compensate for the loss of the outer hair cells by compressing the incoming signals appropriately. It must be noted that for compensation of recruitment, syllabic compression is necessary; this means extremely rapid activation of the compression (attack time < 10 ms; release time < 50 ms). The disadvantage of such rapid adjustment is distortion in the low frequencies. The frequency range to be compressed must be subdivided into various bands, allowing fast attack and release times in the high frequencies and slower ones in the low frequencies where distortions may otherwise occur.

10.4.5 Summation of loudness

The sensory cells (one row of inner and three rows of outer hair cells) are arranged along the basilar membrane such that pitch is perceived at a quite specific point. For this reason, 24 filter bands have been defined along the cochlea. These are the so-called critical bands which have a band breadth of 1 bark. Below 500 Hz, the critical bands are 100 Hz wide. Above 500 Hz, they are divided roughly into one third octave bands.

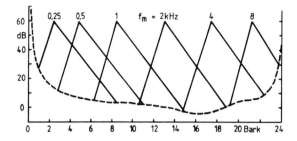

Fig. 10.5: The critical bands according to Zwicker [15]

Fig. 10.5 shows a simplified diagram of the excitation pattern in various bands (adapted from Zwicker; Psychoakustik 1982 [15]). The form of the filters is identical in all critical bands at first approximation.

A pure tone is the simplest of all signals, constituting just one single spectral line. Nevertheless, a pure tone generates a wide excitation pattern on the basilar membrane, spreading over several critical bands as shown in Fig. 10.5. A broad band noise stimulates all critical bands equally. The more critical bands have been stimulated, the greater is the sensation of loudness. For example, if a 1 kHz pure tone at 64 dB SPL and a broad band noise of the same intensity are presented to a listener, the broad band noise will be experienced as being 12 dB more intense.

The explanation for this effect lies in the fact that, with broad band stimulation along the basilar membrane, many more nerve cells are simultaneously contributing to the loudness. Spectral components of a sound lying within a critical band add together physically in accordance with their level; components falling in another critical band experience a greater rating, something which is described in psychoacoustics as summation of loudness. However, summation of loudness decreases for the most part with increasing severity of the hearing impairment and even disappears completely in certain patients. This is because the critical bands widen so that fewer are active than is the case with normally hearing persons. To compensate for decreased or absent summation of loudness, it must be assessed at the diagnosic stage.

At present, selective amplification is determined on the basis of the hearing threshold or with loudness scaling. However, these are both methods based on narrow band stimuli and thus do not reflect any summation of loudness. As a result, broad band signals are experienced as being too loud or narrow band ones too weak. The same problem also arises in the case of maximum output SPL. The maximum output SPL control must depend on the signal spectrum and the summation of loudness so that valuable hearing instrument dynamics do not unnecessarily fall victim to a fitting compromise.

The digital hearing instrument can be made to measure the signal spectrum and thus constantly adapt the frequency-dependent amplification and the maximum output SPL control on the basis of total loudness.

10.4.6 Masking

In Fig. 10.6, the masking curves of a narrow band noise with a center frequency of 1 kHz are shown for various intensity levels. Any pure tone located below such a masking curve will be covered (masked) by the narrow band noise and, thus, not heard. In connection with this, the terms premasking and postmasking are used. Premasking means that a tone below the center frequency of the noise is masked, while postmasking refers to the masking of a signal with a higher frequency than that of the center frequency.

Masking curves are asymmetrical, spreading more on the high frequency side of the center frequency than on the lower side. As a result of this, a low frequency sound disturbs speech understanding to a greater extent than does a high frequency sound because it interferes more with hearing the high frequency components of speech.

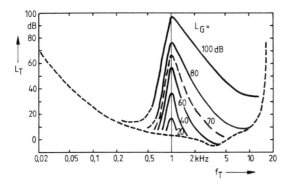

Fig. 10.6: Masking curves of a person with normal hearing

The masking curves are dependent on the level of the masker: with increasing level they become increasingly asymmetrical due to the nonlinear regulating mechanism on the cochlea (through the outer hair cells) only being active at low levels and saturated at high levels. The masking curves run practically uniformly through all critical bands. In the case of hearing impairment, the critical bands widen, and masking curves flatten out and spread upward at much lower levels than is the case with normal hearing.

What are the possibilities for demasking by means of a hearing instrument? As a result of wider masking curves, a hearing-impaired person's perception of the high frequency components of the speech spectrum are hampered to an even greater degree by the low frequency parts of the signal. At present, hearing instruments do not, for the most part, contain any mechanisms for demasking. Adaptive filters in the bass range, or two-channel AGC systems can be somewhat helpful in the case of dominant low frequency interference. However, the algorithms utilized in these instruments compensate for the upward spread of masking by means of steeply sloping filters in the low frequencies. The frequency response curve of such an instrument is consequently steeper than indicated for the individual hearing loss. Wearers often react negatively, because the hearing instruments sound too shrill. In a digital hearing instrument, an adaptive filter demasks the spectra based on a model for normally hearing persons; masked spectral components are amplified as much as possible, while at the same time, compensation for loudness changes occurs. However, if the masking curves for an individual are practically flat, even such a method will not help.

Index

Dictionary

ENGLISH	GERMAN	FRENCH
A		
Acoustic filter	Dämpfungselement	Filtre acoustique
Acoustic gain	Akustische Verstärkung	Gain acoustique
Acoustic modification	Akustische Modifikationen	Modification acoustique
AGC circuit	AGC-Schaltungen	Circuit de CAG
Anechoic chamber	Schalltoter Raum	Chambre sourde
Attack time	Einschwingzeit	Temps d'attaque
Audiogram	Audiogramm	Audiogramme
Audio input	Audio-Eingang	Entrée audio
Audiometer	Audiometer	Audiomètre
Audio input accessories	Audio-Zubehör	Accessoire audio
Audio shoe	Audio-Schuh	Sabot audio
A-weighted	A-Bewertung	Pondération A
B		
Background noise	Störschall	Source perturbante
Basic frequency response	Normale akust. Wiedergabekurve	Courbe de reproduction acoustique normale
Basilar membrane	Basilarmembrane	Membrane basilaire
Battery	Batterie	Pile
BiCROS	BiCROS	BiCROS
Body hearing instrument	Taschengerät	Appareil boîtier
Bone conduction	Knochenleitung	Conduction osseuse
BTE (Behind The Ear instrument)	HdO-Gerät (Hinter dem Ohr Gerät)	Contour d'oreille
Button receiver	Einsteckhörer	Ecouteur enfichable
C		
Calibration	Kalibrierung	Calibration
Capacity	Kapazität	Capacité

Carbon hearing instrument	Telephonie-Hörgerät	Aide auditive type téléphonique
Ceramic	Keramik	Céramique
Ceramic microphone	Keramikmikrophon	Microphone céramique
Circuit	Schaltung	Circuit
Class A receiver	Klass-A-Hörer	Ecouteur classe A
Class B receiver	Klass-B-Hörer	Ecouteur classe B
Class D receiver	Klass-D-Hörer	Ecouteur classe D
Cochlea	Cochlea	Cochlée
Compression	Kompression	Compression
Consonant	Konsonant	Consonne
Couppler	Kuppler	Coupleur
Critical bands	Kritische Bänder	Bande critique
CROS	CROS	CROS
Custom made hearing instrument	Custom Made Gerät	Appareil sur mesure

D

Diffuse soundfield	Diffuses Schallfeld	Champs diffus
Digitally programmable hearing instrument	Digital programmierbares Hörgerät	Aide auditive à programmation numérique
Digital signal processing	Digitale Signalverarbeitung	Traitement numérique du signal
Diode compression	Diodenkompression	Compression à diodes
Directional characteristic	Richtcharakteristik	Caractéristique directionnelle
Directional microphone	Richtmikrophon	Microphone directionnel
Distortion	Verzerrung, Klirrfaktor	Distorsion, Taux de distorsion
Dynamic compression	Dynamikkompression	Compression dynamique

E

Ear	Ohr	Oreille
Ear canal, External auditory meatus	Gehörgang	Conduit auditif
Earmold	Otoplastik	Embout

Ear resonance	Ohrresonanz	Résonance de l'oreille
Ear simulator	Ohrsimulator	Simulateur d'oreille
Ear trumpet	Hörrohr	Cornet acoustique
Eyeglass adapter	Brillenadapter	Adaptateur de lunettes
Eyeglass hearing instrument	Hörbrille	Lunette auditive
Electret	Elektret	Electret
Electret microphone	Elektretmikrophon	Microphone à électret
Electromagnetic	Elektromagnetisch	Electromagnétique
End amplifier	Endstufe	Etage de sortie
Environmental noise	Umgebungslärm	Bruit ambiant
Etymotic frequency response	Etymotischer Frequenzgang	Courbe de réponse étymotique

F

Feedback	Rückkopplung	Effet larsen
Feedback suppression	Rückkopplungs- unterdrückung	Réduction de l'effet larsen
Field effect transistor	Feldeffekttransistor	Transistor à effet de champ
Filter function	Filterfunktion	Fonction de filtrage
Fitting	Anpassung	Adaptation
FM system	FM-System	Système FM
Free field measurement	Freifeldmessung	Mesurage en champ libre
Frequency response	Frequenzgang	Réponse en fréquence
Full on gain	Max. Verstärkungskurve	Courbe de gain maximal
Fully digital hearing instrument	Digitales Hörgerät	Aide auditive numérique

G

Gain	Verstärkung	Gain, Amplification
Gain curve	Verstärkungskurve	Courbe de réponse de gain

H

Hair cell	Haarzelle	Cellules ciliées
Hand held microphone	Handmikrophon	Microphone à main

Headphone	Kopfhörer	Casque écouteur
Hearing healthcare professional	Hörgeräteakustiker	Audioprothésiste
Hearing instrument receiver	Hörgerätehörer	Ecouteur d'aide auditive
Hearing instrument measurement	Hörgerätemessung	Mesurage des aides auditives
Hearing instrument type	Hörgerätetyp	Modèle d'aides auditives
Hearing instrument transducer	Hörgerätewandler	Transducteur d'aide auditive
Hearing instrument accessoires	Hörgerätezubehör	Accessoire d'aide auditive
Hearing loss -mild -moderate -severe, profound	Schwerhörigkeit -leichtgradig -mittelgradig -hochgradig	Perte auditive -légère -moyenne -sévère
Hearing threshold	Hörschwelle	Seuil d'audition
HF-Average	HF-Mittelwert	Moyenne HF
Highpass filter	Hochpass-Filter	Filtre passe-haut
Highpass tone hook	Hochton-Winkelstück	Coude passe-haut
Horn	Horn	Cor

I

Inductive	Induktiv	Inductif
Infrared	Infrarot	Infrarouge
Inner ear	Innenohr	Oreille interne
Insertion gain	Insertion Gain	Gain d'insertion
In-situ measurement	In-Situ-Messung	Mesurage in situ
Internal noise	Eigenrauschen	Bruit de fond
ITE (In The Ear instrument)	IdO-Gerät (In dem Ohr Gerät)	Intra-auriculaire

L

Limiter	Begrenzer	Limiteur
Loudness summation	Lautheit-Summation	Sommation d'intensité
Loudspeaker frequency response	Lautsprecher-Frequenzgang	Courbe de réponse du haut-parleur
Lowpass filter	Tiefpass-Filter	Filtre passe-bas

Lowpass tone hook	Tieftonwinkelstück	Coude passe-bas

M

Masking	Maskierung	Masquage
Measuring box	Messbox	Caisson de mesure
Measurement	Messung	Mesurage
Mercury battery	Quecksilber-Batterie	Pile au mercure
Method of comparison	Komparationsmethode	Méthode de comparaison
Method of substitution	Substitutionsmethode	Méthode de substitution
Microphone	Mikrophon	Microphone
Microphone tubing	Mikrophonschlauch	Tube de microphone
Middle ear	Mittelohr	Oreille moyenne
Modular hearing instrument	Modulares Gerät	Appareil modulaire

N

Noise	Rauschen	Bruit
Non-linear distortion	Nichtlineare Verzerrungen	Distorsion non linéaire
Norm	Norm	Norme
Notch filter tone hook	Kerbfilter-Winkelstück	Coude coupe bande

O

Omnidirectional microphone	Omnidirektional-Mikrophon	Microphone omnidirectionnel
OSPL 90	OSPL 90 (Output sound pressur level 90)	OSPL 90 (Pression acoustique de sortie pour 90 dB d'entrée)
Output limiting	Ausgangsschalldruck-begrenzung	Limitation du niveau de sortie

P

PC (Personal computer)	PC	PC (Personal Computer)
Peak clipper	Peak-Clipper	Peak-clipping
Perception	Hörempfindung	Perception

Pink noise	Rosa Rauschen	Bruit rose
Pistonphon	Pistonphon	Pistonphone
Polar response	Polardiagramm	Diagramme polaire
Pressure microphone	Druckempfänger	Capteur de pression
Programming equipment	Programmiergerät	Console de programmation
Programming	Programmierung	Programmation

Q

Quiescent current	Ruhestrom	Courant de repos

R

Release time	Ausschwingzeit	Temps de retour
Recruitment	Recruitment	Recrutement
Remote control	Fernsteuerung	Télécommande
Resonance	Resonanz	Résonance
Reverberation	Nachhall	Réverbération

S

Saturated sound pressure level	Max. Ausgangs-schalldruckpegel	Pression acoustique max. de sortie
Sound	Klang	Son composé
Sound field	Schallfeld	Champ acoustique
Sound pressure level	Ausgangsschalldruckpegel	Niveau de pression acoustique de sortie
Sound wave	Schallwelle	Onde acoustique
Signal to noise ratio	Signal-Rausch-Abstand	Rapport signal au bruit
Sinusoidal tone, pure tone	Sinuston	Son sinusoïdal, son pur
Speech	Sprache	Parole
Summation	Summation	Sommation
Switch	Schalter	Commutateur
Syllable	Silbe	Syllabe

T

Telephone coil, Induction coil	Telephonspule	Capteur téléphonique
Telephone coil measurement	Telephonspulenmessung	Mesurage de capteur téléphonique
Threshold	Schwellenpegel	Seuil
Threshold of pain	Schmerzschwelle	Seuil de douleur
Tone control	Klangblende	Réglage de tonalité
Tone hook	Winkelstück	Coude
Transducer	Wandler	Transducteur
Transistor	Transistor	Transistor
Tympanic membrane (Ear drum)	Trommelfell	Tympan

U

Ultrasonic	Ultraschall	Ultrason
User control	Bedienungselement	Commande
Uncomfortable loudness level	Unbehaglichkeitsschwelle	Seuil de douleur

V

Vacuum tube	Elektronenröhre	Tube électronique
Venting	Belüftung	Event
Venting	Zusatzbohrung	Event
Vibration sensitivity	Vibrationsempfindlichkeit	Sensibilité aux vibrations
Volume control	Lautstärkesteller	Potentiomètre de gain
Vowel	Vokal	Vocal

W

White noise	Weisses Rauschen	Bruit blanc
Working current	Arbeitsstrom	Courant de fonctionnement
Working current	Betriebsstromstärke	Intensité de courant de fonctionnement

Z

Zink air battery	Zink-Luft-Batterie	Pile zinc-air

Bibliography

[1]   ANSI S3.22-1987: Specification of Hearing Aid Charakteristics, Standards Secretariat Acoustical Society of America New York 1987

[2]   Berger, K.W.: The Hearing Aid, National Hearing Aid Society, 1984

[3]   B & K: Handbuch, Ohrsimulator Typ 4157, April 1981

[4]   Courtois J., Johansen P., Larsen B., Christensen P. and Beilin J.: "Open Molds". In Hearing Aid Fitting, theoretical and practical views, Jensen J.H. (ed), 13th Danavox Symposium, 1988.

[5]   Ditthardt A.: Detailed Application Notes For The Knowles EP Integrated Receiver. Knowles Elektronics, Inc., Maplewood Drive Italsca, Illinois, January 1990

[6]   Güttner, W.: Hörgerätetechnik, Thieme Verlag, Stuttgart 1978

[7]   IEC Publication 118-0: Hearing Aids. Measurement of elektroacoustial characteristics, Genève 1983

[8]   IEC Publication 118-1: Hearing Aids, Hearing aids with induction pick-up coil input, Genève 1983

[9]   Killion M. C. and Carlson E. V.: A Wideband Miniature Microphone. Paper presented at the 37th Audio Engeneering Society Convention, October 1969, New York

10]   Killion M. C. and Carlson E. V.: A Subminiature Elektret-Condenser Microphone of New Design. Paper presented at the 46th Audio Engeneering Society Convention, September 1973, New York

[11]   Knowles Electronics: Directional Hearing Aid Microphone-Application Note, Technical Bulletin TB 21.

[12]   Knowles Electronics: Datasheet Miniature Microphones and Miniature Receivers

[13]   Madaffari P.: Directional Matrix Technical Bulletin. Project 10554, Indrustrial Research Products, Inc. A Knowles Company Report 1983

[14]   Veit I.: Technische Akustik, 2. Auflage. Vogel Verlag, Würzburg 1978

[15]   Zwicker, E.: Psychoakustik. Springer, Berlin-Heidelberg-New York 1982

Notes